# ANSWERS . . . AND QUESTIONS

Every week sees more books added to the growing list of works on health and nutrition—a flood of helpful information. Yet even the best and most thorough of them can't meet each reader's *individual* needs fully, and each book may seem to raise more questions than it answers. In LIGHT ON YOUR HEALTH PROBLEMS, Linda Clark provides a "feedback" from her readers—their intelligent, searching questions, answered in candid, authoritative detail.

Whether your main concern is in nutrition, beauty care, disease prevention, or just plain good health, this fact-packed book has news for you—the best new information on each topic, presented by one of today's most respected health writers and researchers.

*Linda Clark's*

# LIGHT ON YOUR HEALTH PROBLEMS

Keats Publishing, Inc.        New Canaan, Connecticut

Light On Your Health Problems

A PIVOT/*Let's* LIVE Book
Published by arrangement with Oxford Industries, Inc.

Copyright © 1972 by Oxford Industries, Inc.

This material previously appeared in *Let's* LIVE Magazine.

All Rights Reserved

Printed in the United States of America
Library of Congress Catalog Card Number: 72-83522

PIVOT/*Let's* LIVE Books are published by
Keats Publishing, Inc., 212 Elm Street
New Canaan, Connecticut 06840

# CONTENTS

# NUTRITION

Q. Somehow it sounds far-fetched to me when so many success stories are attributed to the use of nutrition. Aren't these exaggerated?—B.T., Philadelphia, Pennsylvania

A. I am afraid a question like this is liable to start a riot among those many, many people who have benefitted from incorporating good nutrition into their diet. It is no exaggeration that we are what we eat, and the better the type of fuel we put into our bodies, the better our bodies become. If you have a pet, I am sure you are careful what you feed the animal to keep him strong, healthy, frisky, energetic and bright of eye with a beautiful coat. If people were required to eat as carefully, they would have (and do have) similar results.

A friend stopped by the other day. She and her husband are newcomers to the good nutrition concept and whereas they formerly dragged with fatigue on their old way of eating, they are now bouncing with energy and good looks on their new program.

My friend said, thoughtfully: "You know, this nutrition program is a completely new way of life and I would not trade it for the old way for anything in the world."

She is the rule, not the exception. Thousands who have tried the nutritional way of life agree with her.

Q. I am a newcomer to nutrition. I am beginning to read books by you, Adelle Davis and others, but I am so confused! How do you go about changing your family's eating? My husband is 39 but feels 79. He has all sorts of things wrong with him. His hands and feet hurt, for one thing, and he just got a new job which requires a lot of walking. (There was no choice—he had to take it.) The doctors at a Veterans Administration Hospital think it's some kind of arthritis. They gave him coated aspirin. A foot doctor gave him Indocin, which made him sick, and he almost lost his job. I got him to take a few vitamins but he still eats white bread, drinks pop as well as milk, and eats such junk as candy and snacks. He is very stubborn and hard to change. We have three kids from 11 to 3 and I don't know what to do for them, either. Is it necessary to buy everything at a health store? Financially, this is pretty hard. Also, there are so many brands of vitamins. How can you know what to get? Please don't tell me to ask my doctor. Doctors couldn't care less about nutrition or vitamins. I don't feel so good myself. I'm having eye troubles, for one thing. Please help me. I want to get in on this world of nutrition, which is so fascinating, but I don't know how to begin or how to get my family to go along with it.—Mrs. C.M., Ames, Iowa

A. All of Adelle Davis' books and mine represent the result of years of work to find the information and relay it to you. Catharyn Elwood and Carlton Fredericks and Lelord Kordel and many others have much help to offer, too. Study them all! These books are in health stores, and cheap at the price for the information you get.

Next, invest in the nutrition cookbooks also in the health stores; most are in paperback form now. Agnes Toms, Beatrice Trum Hunter and Adelle Davis have written excellent cookbooks to get you started. They will show you how to use nutritional ingredients in your recipes which can also be delicious. They will give you school lunch ideas for your children and your husband, too, if he takes his lunch.

To be a good shopper, learn to be a good label reader. If a product is loaded with chemicals, don't buy it! You can find some things at supermarkets which are safe: peanut butter, for instance, which is made of peanuts and salt only. There will be other brands, of course, loaded with fillers and chemicals, but label reading will show you the no-no's. For whole grains, cereals and organic, unsprayed, uncontaminated foods, patronize your health store. I know prices seem higher because these products are not mass-produced like those in supermarkets. They are custom-made, so to speak, and like custom-made clothes, are more expensive but are also of greater value. Family after family has told me that as their health food costs went higher at the health food stores, their doctor's bills went down to the lowest of all time. So good food is cheaper than poor health. And it is the fuel which keeps your body in good condition.

As for vitamins, seek the natural brands. They are concentrated food, not chemicals.

Finally, how to convert your family? Don't preach or you will turn them off before you ever get started. Make your changes quietly, without fanfare. Make some whole grain homemade bread as a starter (it is a good food and full of nutrients). If you have a weight problem, one slice of this will be more satisfying than the "empty calories" found in 10 slices of white bread. Avoid white sugar. Use the so-called raw—which at least has a little nutrition in it—and use less and less. Substitute natural honey whenever possible. Use brown rice instead of white. No one will even know the difference, except that they will notice the rice tastes better. Keep your meals simple: A protein every meal, with a fresh green salad, a quick-cooked vegetable, with fruit and/or cheese for dessert for dinner. For breakfast, serve fruit or real juice, not a juice "drink" (those chemicals again). And try the crunchy new dry cereals at health stores in summer (they are wonderful; children ask for seconds), and use a hot, whole grain cereal in the winter. Fix a good lunch, if possible, for all of you. The cookbooks will give you clues. Pretty soon, this way of eating will be a new way of life and, like others before you, your family will begin to feel and look better. Good luck!

Q. Why is there so much disagreement between "experts" on nutrition? It is very disturbing to many of us.—C.P.D., Pittsburgh, Pennsylvania

A. This is a good question and it deserves a good answer. There are several reasons:

1. No one knows *everything* about nutrition. It is too young a science.

2. Nutritionists (or nutrition reporters such as I) can only report information available *at the time they are writing.* The information is coming from the laboratory so fast that what may be the last word today, may be

out of date tomorrow. This is why many of us document our source *with the date*. It is a full-time job trying to keep up with the avalanche of information, believe me.

3. Why are the findings often different? Many tests are conducted under different circumstances or on animals only. Some animals react as people do, but even different species of animals differ. For example, some manufacture their own vitamin C, others do not. Vitamin C tests would be different in those who manufacture C as compared with those who don't. There are many other possible and similar discrepancies, too.

4. There is another very important reason for disagreement. Often only a single nutrient is tested. Since, in nature, vitamins and minerals work together as a team, the results from testing a single factor might not yield the same results of those nutrients found in combination. And far too often, too low a potency is tested, resulting in disappointing effects. This happened to vitamin E. The amount tested was too low to achieve convincing results, so many doctors rejected it. Also, sometimes not enough time is given for results.

5. Last, but not least, sometimes false or misleading news reports are given out for a drug or a vitamin because the information is "slanted" for commercial purposes. A company may try to attract buyers on one hand, or on the other, discourage buyers because another product is competitive. Even, in some cases, well-known personalities in high places are paid to give misleading information by one or more industries which are trying to sell products. There are proven cases where this has already happened, and as you have witnessed for yourself in many TV commercials, such practices are still continuing.

Q. If you take supplements, does it really matter whether or not you eat carefully?—L.A., San Jose, California

A. The right food is a *must*, even if you do take supplements. Both are necessary, according to Ruth K. Leverton, Ph.D. She reported a survey of the diets of older people in one city in which the diets of one-half of the group would have been improved in nutritive value by the *right* supplements. About one-fourth of these people used supplements which provided *none* of the nutrients that were in short supply in their diets; and one-fourth used supplements that provided some, but not all, of the nutrients which were in short supply.

Not only is proper food the best source of nutrients because it provides factors important to well-being, some of which have not been discovered, or isolated, but food also supplies energy as well as a base for the vitamins and mineral supplements you take with it. (Supplements are better assimilated when taken with food, because, after all, they are food factors.)

Ruth Leverton points out that chemically purified or synthetic foods are not the answer, any more than synthetic isolated vitamins or minerals. For overall good nutrition, a varied diet of wholesome organically raised foods, plus whole natural supplements (derived from food), comes closest to supplying all the factors the body needs to help keep it in good repair.

Q. I am at my wit's end. I have tried to change over to the nutritional way of life. For five years, I have included as many health foods as possible in my cooking. I have also given my family more vitamins. I breast-fed my baby. Result? We all feel worse. Breast milk is supposed to protect babies from cold. Mine gets the sniffles. Vitamin C is supposed to stop colds. We have never had vitamin C stop a cold in this family. What in the world is wrong? Everyone else writes how health foods and supplements have improved their health. Not this family!—M.G., Glendale, California

A. Something is undoubtedly wrong, since your family is the exception, not the rule. Let's see if we can spot the trouble. Are you sure you are reading thoroughly and widely, not just snatching an idea here, another one there? A little knowledge can sometimes be a dangerous thing. About vitamin C for colds, for example. In my experience I have never seen massive doses of vitamin C stop a cold. It may lighten it, or shorten its duration, but I have never seen it STOP one. I have, however, seen vitamin C *prevent* a cold again and again, providing medium-sized doses are taken continuously, assuring a high level in the bloodstream at all times to prevent an infection. I have also seen vitamin C abort a cold IF massive doses are taken at the *first* symptom! The minute a scratchy throat, sneezing, or whatever your characteristic sign of an oncoming cold begins, is the time to start intensive vitamin C therapy with the thousands of milligrams, and often I have witnessed, and experienced, a cold stopped in its tracks.

Next about breast milk. Breast milk has changed with the times, like everything else. It is still the best source of food for a baby, but it, like everything else, reflects the times and what you, the mother, are eating or feeling. Breast milk can be full of DDT if you eat it in your non-organic foods. Do you smoke, take drugs or aspirin? If so, you are feeding, second hand, such contaminants to your baby. Are you tense? If so, so is your baby.

As for the rest of your family, although the health ingredients in cooking are good, what about your supplements? Are they balanced? Are you taking too many or too few? Are they natural or synthetic? Are your foods really organic? Do you read labels when you buy supermarket foods so that you are not cooking with additives and chemicals galore? Are you, perhaps, trying to save money by not going to the health store?

Are you giving all of your family the same supplements in the same amounts, although each may have a different need? A young married woman I know thought she was giving her family the best in food and supplements. They all came from the supermarket, including synthetic supplements. She has had one retarded child and her own health is failing before she has turned 30.

Finally, what about your home atmosphere? Are you preaching and forcing your family to eat and take what you think is good for them? Don't. Provide good food, but keep still about it. They will resist you all the way otherwise, and not digest what they eat. Is there tension and resentment in the family rather than love, harmony, tolerance, forgiveness? Tension can cancel out the effect of the best diet in the world!

Analyze your situation honestly and keep reading and learning. We can't all be perfect, but we can try to improve at whatever stage we find ourselves.

Q. Which is really better, eating a few big meals a day, or eating more small meals more often? Is there any proof that one method is better than the other?—G.S., New Orleans, Louisiana

A. Yes, there is a difference between the effects of eating two or three large meals a day as compared with "nibbling" small meals more frequently, even though the total amount of food eaten may be the same. A study conducted at the Department of Pharmacology, State University of New York, and reported in the *American Journal of Clinical Nutrition*, August, 1970, supplies proof that frequent small meals are better than fewer large ones because energy is supplied as it is needed and helps the body metabolize or *use* the food better than when supplied in larger amounts which are usually eaten in the evening. Serum cholesterol also declined in patients who ate eight small meals a day. Furthermore, the cholesterol-lowering effect of corn oil was found to be more marked if divided between eight small meals. Glucose tolerance was also better in frequent smaller meals. Larger meals were also found to contribute to overweight as well as ischemic heart disease and thicker skin folds.

Thus the recommendation is made that it is better for overall health, as well as maintaining the desired weight, to divide the total amount of food, chosen for an all-around good diet, into six to eight meals and distribute them throughout the day. Or, if this is inconvenient, it is better to have a large, wholesome breakfast to carry one through the day with more energy and a small evening meal. Those who say they aren't hungry enough for a large breakfast, according to these researchers, eat too much the night before.

Q. We are now convinced that we must improve our diet and avoid eating so much processed food. However, we have a very low income and the price of organic foods as well as vitamin-mineral supplements is high. How can we get healthful, raw, organic food, as well as a high protein content into our diet on a modest budget?—P.B., Big Sur, California

A. If you could have a small organic garden, this would supply, at low cost, some fresh vegetables. But there is still another way: Eat a mixture of raw, whole grains. These can be used as a cereal for breakfast or a main dish at other meals. Dr. William D. Kelley, of Texas, says: "Mix together in a large container one pound of each of the following grains and nuts—wheat berries, buckwheat, rye and oat groats, millet, sesame, brown rice, flax, corn (or popcorn), alfalfa, lentils, mung beans, and almonds. (All are available at health stores.)

"Store in refrigerator. Each night, take three or four tablespoons of this mixture and grind it well in a seed mill, or perhaps a blender. Then, just cover with cream or water. Allow to stand at room temperature overnight. Just before eating, add fruit and/or honey to your taste. This is to be eaten raw, not cooked, and should be used daily."

This is a powerhouse of vitamins and minerals. Friends of mine have started this low-cost, high-health regime. They take equal parts of the 14 grains mentioned and mix up in a quart jar. The remainder they keep in a cool place. They started out adding diced apples as the fruit and changed as other fruits came into season. They are delighted with this nourishing food.

Q. I have read that one should not eat bread, potatoes or any other starch or carbohydrate in the same meal with meat. Does this statement have any scientific truth?—D.Z., St. Louis, Missouri

A. Strangely enough, there are two researchers with the same name who have written on this same subject. One, Daniel Munro, M.D., in his books (now out of print), cites many of his cases who have achieved relief from various symptoms by *not* mixing protein with carbohydrates. Then along comes another researcher, H. N. Munro, who states that his detailed research shows that carbohydrate helps protein to be better assimilated! (*Physiological Review,* 1951, 31, 449).

Long ago I remember hearing a statement to the effect that in the meat-and-potatoes diet, there was value in the potatoes helping the digestion of meat. The latter Munro supports this statement.

This is the type of problem that understandably upsets so many people who are trying to learn nutritional facts: that authorities disagree. The only suggestion I have is that perhaps the whole story has not been learned as yet—and perhaps another factor will emerge later to clear up the mystery. Meantime, try to learn what seems to agree best with you. The same shoe size cannot fit us all.

Q. I have heard it is possible to tighten teeth with good nutrition. I have two loose teeth. Does massaging gums with the finger help? Please give any information you can.—Mrs. E.B., Miami, Florida

A. Nutrition is not limited to the body, you know. It includes the mouth, the head, the eyes, the ears, the skin, the hair—the works! Therefore, loose teeth point to poor gums, which should hold the teeth firmly in place. Poor gums are connected with and supply a clue to the rest of the tissues in the body which you can't see. This means that the entire body is showing signs of nutritional neglect. Healthy gums are pink and firm, not red, spongy and bleeding at the slightest touch. Massaging them helps the circulation, but this is putting the cart before the horse. The blood that you circulate to the gums should be full of repair materials to make the gums—and the rest of your body—healthy.

The first requirement is vitamin C. This means not only ascorbic acid, but the whole C family, known as the bioflavonoids, which help to strengthen tissue. But more than that, vitamins A, B, and minerals should be delivered regularly to those gums to firm them up. Far better than finger massage is eating crunchy foods which massage and exercise those gums at the same time. Raw nuts, sunflower seeds, raw vegetables, whole grains, are helpful. Raw fruits, apples in particular, at the end of the day, are even better than a toothbrush, according to Fred D. Miller, D.D.S., the dentist-author of that wonderful little book, *Open Door to Health*. He has saved many a mouthful of teeth, and improved gums by good nutrition alone. Carbohydrates are OUT! Poor gums have been found to be a direct reflection of too many carbohydrates. Sugars and sweets are sticky and cling to the teeth, causing cavities; carbohydrates are soft, pappy-type foods, which require no effort from the teeth and gums. They are pre-chewed, as it were. And last, but most certainly not least, is plenty of protein! Our flesh and tissues are made of protein. If you don't eat enough, the strength and firmness of the body tissues can eventually break down.

In other words, not only are you what you eat, but your mouth, teeth and gums are a dead giveaway of what you are not eating. So get busy, step up your nutrition, making your diet at least 50 percent raw and turn your back on the valueless carbohydrates. Then give your body and your gums time to recover.

Q. As a bachelor I spend little time in my kitchen, and have been getting my vegetables by making a big salad of still-frozen loose-bagged mixed vegetables (carrot cubes, peas, green beans and corn) with safflower mayonnaise. To what extent have these vegetables lost vitamins, minerals, enzymes and nutrients?—J.B., Hollywood, California

A. Although frozen foods have less loss of nutrients than some other types of processed foods (canning in particular), there is always some loss resulting from any form of processing. In freezing, the fresh food is blanched quickly in boiling water before being submerged in cold water to stop further nutrient loss. This immersion in water leaches out some water-soluble vitamins, such as B and C. Also, the longer the frozen food is stored, the greater the nutrient loss. There are innumerable studies of this loss on record and it differs in each type of vegetable. This does not mean we should avoid frozen foods, because they *are* a great improvement over old methods of food preservation. But it does mean that we should not depend upon *any* processed food for our complete nutrition. Raw food, if it is fresh, should be used as much as possible. Many authorities believe 50 percent of our diet should be raw to help protect our health through natural nutrients. Except for fresh fruit, raw vegetable salads are the best means of procuring these natural nutrients, as well as the enzymes which abound in raw food and are the body's house cleaners. Raw salads are also delicious and I know of no nutritionist who does not recommend a raw salad daily.

In the area where you live, you have the privilege of obtaining raw, organic foods the year around. Make the most of it! Buy fresh, crisp lettuce, tomatoes and cucumbers, peppers, radishes, and make a delectable salad daily. Break the ingredients into bite-sized pieces; add oil, some lemon juice or wine vinegar and seasoning if you wish. Toss all together in a large wooden bowl. Take the time for it! You may add five minutes longer daily in your kitchen, but you'll be adding years to your life.

# FOOD ADDITIVES, CHEMICALS AND PESTICIDES

Q. What can you tell us about the BHA and BHT used in oils, even those which claim to be cold-pressed and "containing no preservatives"?—A.T., Hollywood, California

A. The combination of BHA-BHT-Propyl gallate, usually found in oils, is as closely guarded a secret as the effects of cyclamates and The Pill were for so long. Reason: When the public becomes aroused by the danger of a product, profits drop for the manufacturers. In the *Consumer Bulletin,* October, 1961, and August, 1962, issues, in "The Case of the Butylated Twins," hopefully in your library, you will find that no information requested from the U.S. Government from consumers was made available until it was demanded! Then a very diluted report was issued that the twin preservatives produced toxic effects on animals. At that point the government clammed up.

However, in *Let's LIVE* (December, 1969, p. 77) Ann Druffel wrote an article about the preservatives and told of the hard time she had acting as a detective in order to find incriminating evidence. But because she was already aware that these preservatives are added not only to oils but to every breakfast food except grapenuts, as well as potato chips, corn chips, chewing gum, iced tea mix, crackers, roasted peanuts—you name it, it's got it—Ann Druffel did not rest until she found out what truth was available. She did learn that in laboratory tests it caused blind or eyeless offspring in rats, and other researchers found it too toxic for human use, particularly in the liver. It has also been found to reduce the action of three important body enzymes needed to protect health.

The British do not allow the BHA-BHT twins to be used for infant food, and only half the usual amount for adults, but there is no such thing as a safe amount of poison. It can multiply by eating various products containing the offending substance and thus add up to a large dose. When I read labels, BHA and BHT are the first additives I look for. If the food contains either or both, I don't buy it. I am afraid to take the chance.

Q. Is sorbic acid bad? I notice that it is used as a preservative in several varieties of cheese. Perhaps those who read the labels will confuse it with ascorbic acid.—Mrs. A.W.H., Fallbrook, California

A. You are so right! Many people do snap it up, thinking that the terms "sorbic acid" and "ascorbic acid" are the same. Not so! Sorbic acid, also known as potassium sorbate, is a preservative or additive. In a study with rats given sorbic acid in their drinking water, there were no ill effects from one sample of sorbic acid. But in another sample of sorbic acid, also added to the drinking water, two rats developed tumors within 66 weeks, and all the rats had died in 78 weeks. This same type of sorbic acid added to oil and fed to rats produced malignant tumors in five out of six rats (*British Journal of Cancer,* 1968, 22, pp. 762-768). The question is, how are we to know which sorbic acid is safe? Better settle for something else.

Q. My children like hot dogs, but I understand that the kind you get at the supermarket have undesirable additives. Is this true?— C.T., Fresno, California

A. This is absolutely right. You will find that if you read labels on any brand of frankfurters in the supermarkets you will find both sodium nitrate and sodium nitrite have been added. (Sodium nitrite is a similar preservative.) There has been a cloak of secrecy hiding the bad effects of these additives from the public for too long. Recently, however, the truth came to light on one of them, from FDA warnings about two brands of meat tenderizers, which they consider a "potential hazard to health." These tenderizers, according to the FDA, contain about 97 per cent sodium nitrate, as compared with only a small amount included in other tenderizers. The FDA admitted that "in high concentrations sodium nitrate can disrupt the blood's ability to carry oxygen and combine with stomach acids to form a potent cancer-causing agent."

Most poisons can become cumulative in the body so even a "little bit" is unwise. Read labels on sausages and luncheon meats. You will find sodium nitrate and sodium nitrite there, too. Sodium nitrite has even been used in baby foods.

There are limited supplies of frankfurters without these additives in some health stores, if you are lucky enough to find them. Encourage your health store to stock them.

To replace meat tenderizers containing *any* sodium nitrate, buy the kind in the health store which is made from a natural plant tenderizer: papaya.

Q. What is polysorbate 60? I find it listed on the labels of various foods. Is it safe to eat?—T.J., San Diego, California

A. Polysorbate 60 is one of the many non-nutritive additives allowed in foods. It is classified as a surfactant, which is an "anti-foaming emulsifier or dispersing agent." It is found in candies, soft drinks, dill pickles, ice cream, cream whip, cakes, bread and rolls. The FDA claims that in the permitted amounts, this additive is safe. However, Dr. William Hueper, former head of the government's Environmental Cancer Section of the U.S. Public Health Services, states in his book, co-authored with W. D. Conway, *Chemical Carcinogens and Cancers,* that surfactants are not safe. He writes: "In experiments with animals, it has been shown that some chemicals of this type exert carcinogenic (cancer-causing) or weakly carcinogenic effects . . ."

He adds: "Several thousand different chemicals and chemical mixtures used as additives and pesticides for a greater variety of purposes are now incorporated into foods. Many of these have not been adequately tested for carcinogenic properties."

There is little escape from these and other additives which include emulsifiers, mold retardants, anti-oxidants, artificial colors and flavors, chemical preservatives and many more. There are two steps you can take for protection: Continue to read labels and reject a food if it contains any chemical. Another alternative is to write the manufacturer and complain. This was successful in removing a freshness preserver, BHT (a relative of BHA) from a breakfast cereal. Ruth Winter tells in her book, *Poisons in Your Food* (Crown Publishers), of a girl whose throat swelled on a single serving of cornflakes. The doctor finally traced the trouble to BHT in the cereal she ate.

Q. This morning when I opened a fresh can of pineapple juice, I noticed that the inside of the can had patches as if the metal had eroded. My husband complained of a metallic taste in the juice. I called a food processing consultant, and was told that this process is expected, preserves the vitamin C and makes the juice more palatable! I was assured that though the coating was wearing off on the inside of the can, the amount of metal is harmless.—L.P., San Francisco, California

A. I sent your letter across the United States to Beatrice Trum Hunter, who is an expert on poisons in our foods. Here is her answer: "Actually there is very little tin in tin cans. It is used to solder the joints of the cans. However, there are instances of it contaminating the food in improper canning. Tin is poisonous. Other can linings are not good either. Dr. Theron Randolph, the allergy specialist, found that some of his patients could not tolerate food from cans because of the can linings.

"One of the recent problems with can linings has been linked with the nitrate problem. The nitrate, if in high amounts, which is now added to vegetables—including spinach—creates special problems of interaction with the metal linings of cans. As for aluminum cans, aluminum interacts with acid, alkaline, and salt foods."

This explains why Alan H. Nittler, M.D., advises his patients not to use any foods in cans.

Q. I am a grandfather concerned about the diet of my own as well as others' grandchildren. When I look at the labels on prepared baby foods I am horrified at the additives they contain. I hear that sodium nitrate and sodium nitrite have been used in many (read the labels on frankfurters for older children, too). Even table salt, refined white sugar and monosodium glutamate are used in foods for small babies. One company has suspended the use of MSG, but other companies apparently have not. What can we do to protect the future generation?—D.S., Los Angeles, California

A. The man who wrote this letter took the first positive step by enclosing a letter of complaint to one of the major baby food manufacturers. If enough people voice objections, the manufacturers *will* listen. After all, these firms want to make money and they can make it with good foods as well as with bad.

Another method for health-minded mothers of small babies is to skip prepared baby foods and make them themselves. I know several mothers who put the fresh foods, cooked for the family, in a blender and provide flavorful undercooked, unprocessed foods that the babies prefer to the canned variety. Use your noggins, mothers!

Q. I know that the cyclamates are unsafe sweeteners. How about good old saccharin? Isn't it all right to use?—B.H., Indianapolis, Indiana

A. I am sorry to disillusion you about "good old saccharin." For years health exponents were suspicious about it, but the only thing they could find against it, in absence of studies, was that it was a coal-tar product. At last a study has been conducted, using it on mice at the University of Wisconsin. George T. Bryan, Ph.D., has reported that saccharin pellets implanted in urinary bladders of mice produced cancer in many mice tested. Dr. Bryan suggests that the U.S. Department of Health, Education and Welfare should immediately halt the use of saccharin for people who do not need it.

The FDA is arranging other tests of saccharin at the National Cancer Institute in Bethesda, Md., reports to be made within a few months' time. In light of the reversed ban on cyclamates, though they, too, were found unsafe, it will be interesting to learn the announced results of the FDA study on saccharin.

For a saccharin substitute try small amounts of natural honey.

Q. First we hear that pesticides are to be banned, and the next day we hear that they aren't. Meanwhile, can't we protect ourselves by washing fresh foods carefully?—O.D., Houston, Texas

A. You cannot clean all pesticides from fresh foods. Washing fruit removes about a third of the chemical, but as much as two-thirds penetrates the skin or pulp. According to the U.S. Public Health Service, pesticides can be harmful to liver, spleen, kidneys and spinal cord. Dr. Malcolm Hargraves, of the Mayo Clinic, believes that heavy doses of pesticides in humans can lead to leukemia, aplastic anemia, jaundice, and Hodgkins Disease. Let us all urge a complete and immediate ban of all hydrocarbon pesticides.

Q. Will you please comment on Co-salt, a salt substitute? Some of us women want to know what it is made up of.—Mrs. E.C. McE., Kelso, Washington

A. The ingredients of this salt substitute are: choline bitartrate, potassium chloride, ammonium chloride, potassium glutamate, silica, tribasic calcium chloride phosphate. Not to be used without consulting a physician, says the label.

Q. I can't always afford to buy fresh organic fruits and vegetables. Do you know of a solution with which pesticides can be washed off sprayed crops?—A.M.J., Astoria, New York

A. Pesticides which reach the soil become embedded there and are taken up internally by the fruit or plants. Therefore, that type of contamination cannot be washed off. However, in addition, there is often a residue of spray (sometimes visible, sometimes not) on the surface of the food. There are several approaches. Soaking root crops in vinegar-water helps. For such foods as lettuce and celery, in which spray residue may be deeply embedded in the layers or folds, or for any food to which spray clings tenaciously there are several biodegradable liquid soaps which can be added at the rate of 1 to 2 tbsps. per dishpan full of water for soaking.

Q. You say that washing fruit removes only about one-third of the pesticides. I have been told that by adding two tablespoons of vinegar to a pan of cold water, you can remove most of the chemicals from fruits and vegetables, except for Brussels sprouts, artichokes and strawberries. Please comment.—F.H., Las Vegas, Nevada

A. Vinegar in water has been used quite effectively for removing some of the pesticides. The produce is soaked in the solution for a short time to help loosen the pesticides, then rinsed off with clear water. Two tablespoons of salt in a pan of water has also proved helpful. Both solutions are used in foreign countries where bacteria count of raw foods is high. The reason that Brussels sprouts, artichokes and strawberries are excepted is the many-layered manner in which they grow. (Lettuce is another example.) Spraying is done successively as the plants mature and the pesticides are trapped inside of the overlapping leaves. Strawberries, because of their "pock-marked" texture, apparently also release the pesticides grudgingly. But whatever the method of washing the surface of the food, the pesticide which is built in from the soil becomes a part of the plant and cannot be removed.

Q. The labels on cartons of ice cream in the supermarkets state only that pasteurized milk and artificial coloring is used. Can you tell me what other ingredients are used?—S.P., San Anselmo, California

A. For flavorings found in the supermarket ice creams, you will find a list of their sources in my book, *Stay Young Longer.* Be prepared for some shocks! Also, a nutrition expert recently told me that there were more illnesses from artificial flavorings and colors, including those in ice cream, than the general public realizes.

From *The National Observer,* as reprinted in the *National Health Federation Bulletin,* Feb., 1970, comes this information on ice cream: "Ice cream comes as close to being completely synthetic as it legally can . . . The minimum standards have finally been set by the FDA after 24 years of government-industry bickering. A gallon of ice cream must now weigh at least 4½ pounds; it may have 100 per cent over-run, meaning a manufacturer can inflate a gallon of mix into 2 gallons of ice cream, including half again as much air as found in premium ice creams (which are not found in the average supermarket).

"The standards include a generous list of such arcane natural products as agar-agar, algin, carageenan (all seaweed products) gum acacia, guarseed gum, gum karaya, locust bean gum, and oat gum (all from plants). It gives its blessing to such chemical additives as propylene glycol (the anti-freeze constituent), glycerin, sodium carboxy-methylcellulose, and it permits the use of disodium phosphates, tetrasodium pyrophosphate, polysorbate 80, and dioctyl sulfosuccinate.

"Most of these additives are used as 'stabilizers' and 'emulsifiers.' Stabilizers make ice cream smooth; emulsifiers make it stiff so it can retain air (most low-priced ice cream contains as much air as it does ice cream). There are other synthetics and substitutes such as corn syrup (instead of sugar or honey), dried eggs (instead of fresh), vanillin (instead of vanilla). As for flavor, it is possible to create boysenberry ice cream without boysenberries, and maple pecan without maple syrup and without pecans. Most important, these substitutes make it possible to cut manufacturing costs.

"Top grade ice cream contains cooked syrups, heavy custards, salt, fresh eggs, fresh cream, sometimes gelatin. Flavorings include such things as vanilla beans, pure chocolate, and fresh fruits. It also contains air—a necessary ingredient that enters the mix when it's whipped."

Unfortunately, the FDA does not require the exact ingredients to be stated on the label so the average consumer is buying blind. Fortunately for those of us who live in California, we can buy at health stores ice cream made from certified raw milk and cream, honey and natural flavorings, just like Grandma used to make, and the likes of which modern children will never taste again—unless you make your own!

Q. I have discovered some packages of freeze-dried food with ingredients for chicken and beef casseroles, etc., on the grocer's shelf. Is this acceptable for eating?—H.G., Miami, Florida

A. I asked this same question of Agnes Toms several years ago and she gave freeze-drying her O.K. Knowing Mrs. Toms' reputation as an expert in the field of cooking and nutrition, and being an admirer of her cookbook, *Eat, Drink and Be Healthy* (in paperback at health stores), her word is enough for me. However, here is more scientific reassurance for doubting Thomases. In a German study, freeze-drying, compared with other drying processes at normal pressure or under vacuum, was found not to change most food products chemically. The foods which were freeze-dried retained their normal appearance, flavor and odor and could be easily reconstituted (Nahrung, 1967, 11, 267-276). For a while freeze-dried food was available mainly in camping supply outlets. No doubt it is being used for space flights. Only recently is it becoming available in some grocery stores. I have not tried it yet. According to labels, several varieties have added preservatives, but one, using chicken, does not, and may be worth trying.

Q. At least one physician insists that fluorides are effective for treatment of osteoporosis. This physician contends that adding fluorides to the water supply is therefore beneficial. Is it true or false that fluorides help osteoporosis sufferers?—D.B., Boston, Massachusetts

A. Osteoporosis is a form of atrophy of the bone without it changing shape. Some people call it a "softening" of the bone. At any rate, it reduces the bone mass to the point where it is below the level of mechanical support. It is usually thought to be related to a calcium deficiency. An answer to your question has appeared in the respected *American Journal of Clinical Nutrition*, in the January, 1971, issue. A study conducted by four physicians at Medical Research Center, Brookhaven National Laboratory, Long Island, New York, revealed the following information: There was a slight increase of calcium as a result of fluoride supplementation, but after two to seven months of fluoride treatment, the total body calcium was not significantly increased. The findings stated: "Based on these results and on clinical observations, fluoride cannot be considered an effective treatment for osteoporosis."

Q. I recently heard a TV star state that he uses tablets made from reindeer liver because there is very little DDT or other pesticide residues where the reindeer live. I would appreciate your comments.—M.G., Miami, Florida

A. I do not like to be a killjoy, but though there may not be much DDT where reindeer live (in the far, far North), there is certainly a lot of fallout. The fallout is not only high in that area, it settles on the lichen which is eaten by the animals who absorb the radiation. I would prefer the DDT to the fallout, because this you can control. One liver product (desiccated liver tablets) available in this country is derived from Argentina, which does have little DDT (although this is now a world-wide problem). However, the best solution of all is to take desiccated liver tablets which are defatted. DDT settles in the fatty tissue, including the liver. If the fat is removed at the low temperature which is used for desiccation, the remaining liver is free of the pesticides. To find defatted liver tablets, read labels at your health stores.

Q. There has been much recent information appearing in the press about the mercury contamination of the waters off the Pacific Coast and other waters. Since sea vegetation is a natural source of trace minerals, is there a potential source of danger to the vitamin and mineral tablets derived from seaweed and fish products? Also, what about the sea water sold in health stores? Is it safe to add to distilled water for mineral content?—R.J.S., North Riverside, Illinois

A. I asked manufacturers of these products whom I know and trust for their opinions. One of them answered: "We have been deeply concerned about this question as well as that of pesticides possibly contaminating products for both animals and humans. Periodically the FDA takes samples of the Pacific Ocean in which some 14 different kinds of sea plants grow. As yet they have found no contamination. The kelp we harvest off the California coast north of Santa Barbara and San Clemente Islands has shown no contamination. With new awareness of the causative factors and better controls, we doubt that we will run into trouble."

A company which provides purified (without heat), filtered sea water says: "Our first test on our sea water showed no traceable amount of mercury present."

As for fish liver oils (a source of vitamin A and D supplements), a recent test made by a company which imports the raw products from all over the world and distributes them to many manufacturers, showed only .02 parts per million of mercury (considered a microscopic amount).

Vitamin/mineral companies really have the interests of their customers at heart. As an example, five years ago one company which processes fish liver oil and at that time received its raw material off the coast of Alaska, which is practically uninhabited, tested and found 60 parts per million of mercury! They promptly took it off the market. Although mercury may well be a world-wide problem, there are areas which are little contaminated (Norway and Nova Scotia, for example), and wherever these safer waters exist, sea products will be taken from them. A recent newspaper article states that actually mercury is not a new problem; it has existed for a long, long time. However, now that the effects are known, its content will be carefully monitored in food in order to protect the public.

# FOODS

## Dairy Foods

Q. What is the best spread to use, margarine or butter?—D.K., Minneapolis, Minnesota

A. I am always shopping around looking for a good margarine which tastes like butter and still has polyunsaturates and as few artificial additives as possible. I asked Beatrice Trum Hunter, author of the *Natural Foods Cookbook*, what she used. She told me, "I use unsalted butter on the table. I add no butter to vegetables. Those who wish to do so can add it at the table. For baking and broiling I use natural corn germ oil or crude soy oil, depending on whether I want a mild or strong flavor. For a butter blend of your own, you might blend ⅔ butter, softened at room temperature, with ⅓ good vegetable oil, and refrigerate. Dr. Ancel Keyes suggests, instead of artificial 'cream' so prevalent in markets today, to use, as a coffee cream, a mixture of skim milk and vegetable oil smoothed in a blender." Whatever product you use, read your labels before buying!

Q. I am very much confused since being told by someone in a health store that margarine causes heart trouble and to buy butter instead. In order to avoid high cholesterol problems, I have been buying safflower margarine. Can you clear this up for me?—D.S., Marina Del Rey, California

A. The reason you were told to buy butter in preference to margarine is that margarine is hydrogenated; whereas the right type of butter is natural, contains a variety of unsaturated fats and melts at body temperature—all facts which were given to me by Frank Lachle, the expert on fats and oils.

Beatrice Trum Hunter apparently is in agreement. In her wonderful new book, *Consumer Beware!*, she points out that margarine labels state that the margarine is partially hydrogenated or hardened (which means the same thing), but she says it is either hydrogenated or it isn't! Any degree of hydrogenation is contra-indicated for health, according to present beliefs. A further description of the problems in connection with margarine is truthfully spelled out in Mrs. Hunter's book. Even the FDA is trying to issue mild warnings about health claims for margarines.

The very fact that margarine is solid, not liquid, proves it is hydrogenated. However, it is also true that there have been studies which showed that some butter has caused a rise in cholesterol. So what can you do? Fortunately, there are two ways out. First, you can eat butter (it must be the right kind) and add lecithin, either in granule or liquid form, to your diet. Lecithin helps to dissolve cholesterol and keep it under control. (Possibly you could use it also, along with margarine, in your diet, for the same reason.)

What type of butter is preferred? Mrs. Hunter suggests that it should be made from sweet cream, and is labeled as such. She prefers that it be sweet butter, and she tells why in her book.

The other solution is to do what Gayelord Hauser does. In an interview in *Vogue*, July, 1971, he tells of a trick taught him by an Italian: Soften a pound of butter, add equal parts of safflower oil; melt butter at gentle heat and re-mix, then refrigerate. Mr. Hauser uses it for his toast as well as for cooking purposes.

Q. I cannot find the number of calories for low fat milk, skim milk or regular homogenized milk. Can you help?—Mrs. J.McC., Berkeley, California

A. A cup of skim milk contains 103 calories; a cup of low fat milk has 134 calories and a cup of regular homogenized milk has 154 calories. But don't go off the deep end and avoid whole milk! Everyone needs some fat and many nutritionists feel that whole milk is a valuable source of it even in reducing. Calories in whole, natural foods (as compared with sweets and other carbohydrates) do not tell the whole story. Overweight (edema), gall bladder disturbance, skin diseases, etc., can result from not having enough of the right kind of fat in the diet. So don't avoid a good food merely because of its calories.

Q. My doctor has told me not to eat eggs, particularly egg yolks, because they contain cholesterol. I don't see how I can get along without eggs, either in eating or cooking. What shall I do?—Mrs. F.W., Indianapolis, Indiana

A. Your doctor is evidently one of those men so busy with his patients that he hasn't had a chance to catch up on his reading. Eggs were at one time falsely condemned for the reasons that he mentions. The story today has been found to be different. A study conducted in 1968 at Highland General Hospital, Oakland, California, found that of 13 persons who took egg yolk fat, the equivalent of 50 to 113 egg yolks daily, only two showed a rise in cholesterol, while the others maintained a normal serum cholesterol. (*Metabolism*, 1968, 17, 1129-1139.) Since I presume you eat only one or more eggs a day, instead of 50 or more, this study shows that you have nothing to worry about.

Q. Please tell me why it is wrong to eat raw eggs. What will it do to my body?—R.S., St. Louis, Missouri

A. There is no reason to my knowledge why anyone cannot eat a raw egg yolk. When raw eggs are fed to animals, the animal coats gain luster as well as good growth. Many people believe they notice allergic symptoms when they eat a raw egg in a milk shake or protein drink, or fruit juice—all common methods of taking raw eggs. This slight disturbance may truly exist, but if it does, it is usually due to the raw egg *white,* not the yolk. Joseph D. Walters, M.D., states that people who are allergic to raw egg white usually have no trouble with a raw *fertile* egg white. (A fertile egg is one which hatches and is considered more nutritious.) Dr. Walters explains that the reason is that the fertile egg white makes cystine, an amino acid, available to the body, whereas the infertile egg white does not. He states that most people are deficient in cystine. Dr. Walters is a nutritional physician and I have great respect for his research.

Q. Is cheese a good source of protein, compared with meat? One author states that meat is a "dead" food. I don't mind this, but what about cholesterol?—A.J., Don Mills, Ontario, Canada

A. Meat, a ¼-lb. serving, contains 15-22 grams of protein. Two slices of cheese contain about 10-15 grams of protein. Both are complete proteins, meaning that all the essential amino acids needed by the body are present. I have covered the subject of protein fully in my book, *Secrets of Health and Beauty* and will not repeat it here. Besides I don't want to start an argument about what kind of protein is best. The body is largely made of protein and nutritionists are in agreement that without enough of it, deterioration of the body gradually takes place in most cases. (There are apparently exceptions to every rule.) Protein from meat is the closest in quality to human protein, and, in the opinion of many, the most valuable. Others, of course, disagree. However, cheese can be a problem. If it is pasteurized, enzyme-wise, it is also "dead." If it is *not* made from certified raw milk, and is unpasteurized, it might cause undulant fever, a vicious, debilitating and long-lasting disease, extremely hard to detect. Doctors tell me undulant fever is on the rise.

The type of protein must be a matter of personal choice after studying the facts intelligently about its needs for and use by the body. One should also choose *any* protein from the safest possible sources. As for cholesterol, its causes are many. It can be managed by using lecithin, which is removed by processing dairy products.

Q. Recently a friend told me that cheese contains rennin, which is obtained from the mucous membrane of the stomach of calves.

Since I am a vegetarian, but have been eating natural cheese from the health food stores, I would like to know whether all cheeses contain rennin?—J.M., Franklin, Wisconsin

A. I checked this question with a raw certified dairy and was told that all hard cheese is made with rennin, which causes the milk to solidify more quickly. However, the dairy (one of the most respected in the United States) said that the membrane of the calf's stomach was not used, but the coagulating *enzyme* which occurs in the gastric juice of the calf, and curdles the milk. This is somewhat similar to the hydrochloric acid in your own digestive system. It supplies acid in order to promote better digestion of proteins and minerals.

Q. I was startled and became indignant the other day when I asked for real whipping cream at the grocery store. The owner, who believes in organic food, told me that to his knowledge, all over the U.S. only synthetic whipping cream is now available, because it lasts so much longer on the shelf. Is this true?—E.B., Monterey, California

A. I was told the same thing. The boxes which are kept in the dairy department of grocery stores and supermarkets look exactly like the original whipping cream boxes and the average housewife reaches for the product without reading the label which reveals that the mixture is loaded with chemicals. According to *Popular Science*, two nutritional scientists, Dr. Elaine R. Monsen and Dr. Ancel Keyes, found that a dozen brands of the "low calorie cream substitutes" contained 20% more saturated fatty acids than the dairy creams they replace. Many of the synthetic creams are made from coconut oil. Dr. Keyes said, "This is the worst oil they could have chosen . . . two times as bad as butter oil on the cholesterol level of the blood."

Half-and-half cream seems to be still available, but whipping cream from the cow is disappearing. Most of us do not use whipping cream every day, but when we want it for a special occasion we want the real thing and not a bunch of chemicals. A friend told me she found one natural brand in an out-of-the-way store, and let's hope there are others. Those are the ones for me!

Q. Can anyone tell me a foolproof recipe for making yogurt without a yogurt maker? I have tried several methods but have never achieved that custardy texture it's supposed to have. I have heated the milk to 115, cooled it to 100, added the yogurt, then put in glass jars and set the jars on hot pads on top of the pilot light on the stove for 4, 6, 8 hours, and it is still runny as milk! I even tried the oven for 3 hours, but it is still runny! I give up. I always use yogurt sold at health stores as the culture, so that's not the trouble.—N.Y., Columbus, Ohio

A. To begin with, the reason for heating the milk to scalding in some recipes is for raw milk only. An enzyme in unheated raw milk prevents it from setting, as raw pineapple juice prevents gelatine from setting. However, if you heat the pasteurized milk to 100 degrees or even slightly less, that cannot be your trouble. I believe it is your method of incubation. I make my mixture as you do, pour it into glass jelly glasses, place them in water in an electric frying pan, cover, turn on the control to slightly under 125 or slightly above 100. In about three hours it has become custard-like. Adding powdered milk to plenty of new yogurt starter also helps. Adelle Davis has a good recipe in her cookbook, *Let's Cook It Right* (at health stores). She uses canned milk, plus powdered milk, plus water. I have other friends who use extra-rich jersey milk and still others who use half-and-half. The latter makes a stiff but delicious custard.

If you do not have an electric frying pan, place your jars on an electric heating pad and cover them with a Turkish towel to maintain a regular temperature. I do believe uncontrolled temperature is your problem.

Q. I want to make yogurt from raw milk but have not been successful. It does not get very thick. My recipe says to scald the milk. Since the milk is raw I want to preserve the enzymes in it by not heating it. I heat the milk to only 115 degrees in an electric yogurt maker—which acts as an incubator. Is my trouble due to lack of sufficient heating?—Mrs. N.H., Castro Valley, California

A. I checked with two experts in this field, one on the nutrition staff of Cornell University. Their answer was in agreement: that one enzyme which causes souring of the milk must be eliminated by scalding in order to make yogurt, but that the other enzymes were not damaged by this amount of heat.

However, in his *No Cook-Book,* John H. Tobe gives directions for making clabber, or thick milk, which he also calls yogurt, without any heating or starter at all. He admits that some people would say that clabber is not the same as yogurt but he, like you, objects to boiling (not scalding) raw milk, which he says kills off all the helpful bacteria. His method: Put any amount of raw milk into a bowl or wide mouthed jar and cover with a thin cloth or paper towel. Set this in a warm place, between 75 and 85 degrees. Stir several times to mix the cream throughout. It usually takes from 30 to 48 hours to thicken. At that time, refrigerate.

Some people have been having problems making yogurt by the regular recipe this summer. The problem was solved when the yogurt was allowed to incubate several hours longer than usual. Friends from India make a similar product to yogurt by adding a starter to milk heated so that one's finger can remain in it with comfort, then removing from heat and covering the container (a heavy crock or iron pot to help hold the heat) with a turkish towel until the mixture sets. They call this "curds." They report that weather and atmospheric condition affect the length of time needed for coagulating even though the recipe is followed precisely each time.

Some people add powdered skim milk (¾ cup to 1-1½ quarts of rich milk) to make a firmer texture. Experiment with your milk and equipment and method until you achieve desired results.

Q. A woman wrote you that she was having trouble making yogurt with raw milk. You gave her your suggestions and I would like to share my method, which is also successful.—Mrs. T.H.A., Gettysburg, Pennsylvania

A. I am delighted to have readers share their helpful experiences in this column. Here is the method given by Mrs. T.H.A.: "I am able to secure raw milk from an organic farmer near my home. I get it only once a week and find it keeps very well in the refrigerator. I secured a styrofoam case used for carrying cold drinks for picnics. Mine holds six glasses with the bottom ridges removed. I am careful to rinse everything I use with very hot water and I fill the glasses with hot water and put them in the case while I am preparing the yogurt.

"Measure 5½ glasses of milk into a saucepan, place a thermometer in it and *slowly* bring the milk to 115°. In the meantime, I place 4 tablespoons of powdered skim milk and ½ glass of yogurt in a bowl and mix until smooth; then dilute it with the milk from the pan which is at 115°. Bring the mixture back again to 115°, fill the glasses with it and close the case. It usually takes 4 to 5 hours, but it doesn't matter, since the case has usually cooled and it's hardly possible to leave it too long. Cover the glasses with foil caps and place in refrigerator. I buy the original yogurt, or culture, at health stores. I do not like to scald the raw milk since it then would be no different than pasteurized. I experimented with this procedure until it was satisfactory. I hope it will be of some benefit to others."

## Grains

Q. We are told that eating uncooked grains is detrimental; that they must be baked or cooked.—Mrs. H.E.M., Hemet, California

A. We do know that uncooked wheat germ is considered very healthful, though less palatable than cooked wheat germ; however, I do not believe uncooked grains are detrimental. Studies using raw oatmeal in the original Swiss cereal, *Muesli,* have shown extremely beneficial results. Boiling water is poured over the oats to warm and thicken them slightly, but they are not cooked. Some people chew wheat berries with no noticeable bad results.

Animals, which have a different type of digestive system than humans, thrive on uncooked grains, but many foods, particularly those high in starch, are not only more palatable in cooked form but are better assimilated. For example, carrots, though acceptable raw, are found to liberate more vitamin A when they are cooked.

Grains of all kinds have been known for centuries and, because many are hard to chew and it is difficult for us to extract the nutrients from them, millers crushed them between two large stones (called stone-ground) to get cereal (if coarsely ground) or flour (if finely ground). Man has had fire for a long time, and bread is mentioned throughout the Bible, so apparently, although fruit, and some vegetables and herbs may have been eaten raw, bread was always cooked. There is also evidence of sun-cooking as well as cooking by fire.

Many people, because of digestion problems, or teeth problems, may not be able to eat a 100 percent raw diet. This is why nutritionists urge that the diet be at least 50 percent raw, and allow for the balance of the diet to be cooked or not according to individual needs.

Q. You have stated the advantages of stone-ground flour over the steel roller method because the steel roller method destroys the structure of the grain, greatly reduces protein and kills B vitamins. What happens to stone-ground flour when the bread is baked in a 350 degree oven, and then toasted?—Mrs. G.B., Wakefield, Quebec, Canada

A. The processes by steel rollers reach a far greater heat and a more prolonged treatment than stone grinding with its comparatively short time of baking in a much lower temperature. There is some loss, of course, and still more loss by toasting, but the end product still contains far more nutrients than that subjected to the steel roller method, and *then* oven baked and possibly toasted. To get a general idea of what flour goes through when treated by the steel roller method, read the statements by Fred D. Miller, D.D.S., concerning the commercial treatment of cereals in general, in my article, "The Truth About Cereals," *Let's LIVE,* Sept., 1970, issue. This proves that, although we do eat bread cooked, it is true that for many foods, the less cooking, the better.

Q. Ever since I read the Choate report that the average breakfast food is deficient in energy-giving nutrients, I have been stumped over what to give my family for breakfast. Can you suggest any cereal which can be eaten cold in any season which really provides nutrients and energy?—F.W., Atlanta, Georgia

A. Although I never did eat the usual cold cereals because of the sugar and chemicals added, still I, too, kept looking for an "energy breakfast" and I have found it. John Tobe, in his book, *Guideposts to Health and Vigorous Long Life,* started me off with a recipe he gives for a highly nutritious and "raw" breakfast. I used the basic idea but made a few changes to suit my own tastes and I am delighted with the flavor (when made as directed) and the resulting energy. Here is my version of Mr. Tobe's recipe:

Mix in a large paper or plastic bag the following ingredients, all available at health stores. The amounts are not too important; whatever is convenient, perhaps a package, or half a package, or whatever you wish. The ingredients include raw oats, rolled or steel cut (if rolled, use the old-fashioned kind, not the instant), pearl barley, rice polishings, brewer's yeast, plus calcium lactate to balance the protein content (¼ cup calcium lactate powder to 1 lb. brewer's yeast), granular lecithin, hulled sunflower seeds, whole flaxseed, raisins and a few chia seeds (a few go a long way). The variations are endless. You may add millet, toasted wheat germ or fresh ground whole wheat *providing* you grind it fresh daily to add as needed to prevent rancidity, or whatever you wish. After mixing all ingredients thoroughly in the bag, transfer to a large container and refrigerate. Make it monthly for quick daily use.

This cereal is served RAW, which is part of its value. You can put dried apricots or other dried fruit at the bottom of each bowl per person, the night before, covering the fruit with boiling water then adding about three tablespoons of the cereal mix and adding more boiling water to cover. Cover the bowl with a saucer. You may also prepare this about an hour before serving in the morning and, if you prefer, you can substitute a fresh sliced apple in the morning, or other fruit in season. (The fresh fruit should not stand overnight.) If you wish sweetening, add a bit of honey, and top with whole milk if you wish. It is a whole meal, loaded with B vitamins and protein.

Q. I have read that baker's yeast is somewhat unhealthy, and likewise baking soda and baking powder. Which is best and which is worst? What about sourdough starter which can be used without either soda or baking powder; is it healthful?—Mrs. H.T.M., San Rafael, California

A. I have never heard that baker's yeast is not healthful, unless it is when it is used raw, in which case it is claimed to feed upon the B vitamins in the intestinal tract, stealing them from the host. Yeast is usually as valuable as the food ingredients on which it is fed, and when it is "killed" by cooking, it still retains that goodness. Soda destroys B vitamins outright in food.

Baking powder varies. Some include additives which most of us try to avoid. I try to use baker's yeast whenever possible, but in some cases, such as in biscuits, I use a cream of tartar baking powder which includes cream of tartar, tartaric acid (the acid of grapes) bicarbonate of soda and starch. This well-known brand appears on every grocery shelf. Read your labels.

Sourdough starter is excellent, particularly when unbleached flour is used. I find that after a while it may need strengthening with a baker's yeast now and then. Sourdough, though cooked (like baker's yeast), is considered healthful and an aid to the intestinal flora.

Q. What does yeast do to bread? I read it wasn't as good for you as unfermented bread. Please explain.—C.T. (no address)

A. I called Agnes Toms on this one. She said that yeast not only helps make bread light, it also produces more volume. Unleavened bread is flat, solid and dense, as well as hard to chew. In addition to providing a lighter texture and adding more volume so that the loaf of bread is much larger, the yeast contains B vitamins which multiply as the bread rises. Although the baking halts this multiplication process, it does leave the increased residue of the B vitamins in the bread, making it more nutritious than it was before the yeast was added. As you probably know, Mrs. Toms has been the food page editor of *Let's LIVE* for many years.

Q. I make my own bread from what I consider a very healthful recipe. It contains whole wheat flour, soy flour, yeast, nutritional yeast (brewer's), wheat germ, honey, powdered milk and oil. Recently someone told me that oil in bread is very bad and that butter should be used instead because, according to this person, when the oil is heated it becomes saturated and then the bread is an incomplete carbohydrate. Now I am really confused, especially since the health food cookbooks use oil in their bread recipes. This same person said I should not heat the powdered milk, either. Please help!—D.G., Aspen, Colorado

A. No wonder you are confused. I am wondering where in the world your adviser picked up this information, or I should say misinformation, since it is all false. I double-checked with experts in nutrition all down the line.

The expert on oils said that heating unsaturated oil does *not* make it saturated; it merely reduces the size of the molecules. Heated or unheated, it still remains unsaturated. It is wise not to heat the oil to the smoking point in a frying pan, because it increases the oxidation which lessens its health value, but it still does not turn it into a saturated fat. However, with normal heating, below the smoking point, and certainly in bread which is baked at a relatively low temperature for oils, there is absolutely no detrimental effect. Furthermore, there is no such thing as an incomplete carbohydrate. There are incomplete *proteins,* not incomplete carbohydrates. And there is nothing wrong with heating powdered milk, either. It has already been heated in the process of turning it from liquid milk into powdered milk, and a little more heat is not going to hurt it. Many people use it in hot drinks, gravies and other heated forms. Adding it to bread is no different. As a matter of fact, the famous Cornell University recipe, known as "Cornell Bread," formulated by Dr. Clive M. McCay, contains unbleached white flour, wheat germ, soy flour and non-fat dry (powdered) milk. Rats eating this bread thrived, as did their children, their children's children, and down to the fourth generation. Rats fed enriched bread became sickly and starved looking. Their children were stunted; *their* children died! Your recipe is an improvement even on this excellent bread and I wish I had a slice fresh from the oven this minute!

Q. Some time ago you wrote about a woman in Colorado who made some healthful bread but was disillusioned by a nutritionally uneducated critic who told her she had done everything wrong. You said this recipe was similar to the Cornell Bread, tested on four generations of rats at Cornell University, with great health benefits and that the critic couldn't have been more wrong. I want that recipe!—Mrs. A.D., California City, California

A. Several people have written asking for this recipe. Here is D.G.'s recipe:

## Diana's Bread

Soften two tablespoons baker's yeast in three cups of warm water.

Add ¼ cup molasses and ¼ cup honey. Mix and let stand.

Sift together, then mix:

6 cups whole wheat flour
½ cup flour
¾ cup dry milk
3 tbsps. wheat germ
2 tbsps. nutritional (brewer's) yeast
2 tsps. salt

Add to yeast mixture:

3 tbsps. oil and one-half of the flour mixture.

Beat well, add the remainder of flour.

Let rise for ½ hour.

Bake at 375° for 50 minutes.

Makes three loaves.

You might also like to have the Cornell recipe which it so closely resembles. Here it is:

*Family Recipe for Cornell (Triple Rich) Bread.* Makes

three loaves. Place in a large bowl and let stand for 5 minutes: 3 cups warm water (85°), two packages of yeast (cake or dry), and 2 tablespoons honey or blackstrap molasses or half-and-half of each (which I prefer).

Mix well: 6 cups unbleached flour, plus 3 tablespoons wheat germ, ½ cup full fat flour and ¼ cup dry skim milk powder.

Stir the yeast mixture, adding 4 teaspoons salt and ½ to ¾ of the flour mixture. Beat vigorously 75 strokes. Add 2 tablespoons vegetable oil. Work remainder of flour in, mix thoroughly, and turn dough on a floured board, using one or more cups of flour as needed.

Knead vigorously about 5 minutes or until the dough is smooth and elastic. Place in a greased bowl, grease top of dough lightly, cover bowl and put in a warm place at about 85° until nearly double in size (about 45 minutes).

Punch dough down, fold over edges and turn upside down in bowl to rise another 20 minutes. Turn onto board, divide into three portions. Fold each toward the center to make smooth tight balls. Cover with a cloth and let stand 10 minutes on the board.

Shape into three loaves, or two loaves and a pan of rolls. Transfer to greased tins or pyrex bread containers about 3½" by 7½". Let rise again until dough is double in size, about 45 minutes. Bake at 350°, about 50 to 60 minutes. If the bread begins to brown in 15 or 20 minutes, reduce temperature to 325°.

Remove bread from pans, put on a rack to cool, and brush with melted butter if desired. Let cool completely before eating, wrapping, storing or freezing.

## Fruits, Juices and Drinks

Q. I love papayas. But are they nutritious? Aren't they high in calories?—J.J., Encinitas, California

A. One cup of cubed papaya contains the following:
   * 70 calories
   * 18 grams of carbohydrates
   * 89 percent water

* 36 grams of calcium; 29 mg. phosphorus
* 102 mg. of vitamin C
* 3,190 I.U. of vitamin A
* Small amounts of B vitamins and iron

Q. How many tablets of desiccated liver do you have to take to equal a serving of fresh liver?—M.B., Richmond, Virginia

A. It depends upon the size and weight of the serving of liver. Ten 10-grain tablets of desiccated liver are the equivalent of one ounce of fresh liver. If your serving is four ounces, it would take 40 tablets to equal this much. However, most people take desiccated liver as a source of B vitamins and other nutrients, either because it is a convenience or because they do not like liver. In some brands, the desiccated liver has been defatted and defibered, thus reducing bulk so that fewer tablets can be taken to provide nutrients. Since DDT is stored in the fat, this defatting process removes such poisons. However, at least one brand is not defatted since this company claims its liver comes from a South American country where pesticides are not used. In this case, the desiccated liver would be whole and natural. I cannot state brand names so please read the labels of these products in your health food store.

Q. In an article published by a health food guide, it said: "Do not use lemon juice—it attacks teeth." Is there any truth in this?—M.S., Montreal, Canada

A. Yes, it is true that citrus juices, particularly lemon juice, can attack and erode the enamel on teeth, but that does not mean that one should avoid it. Even blackstrap molasses and other sticky substances, particularly sweet ones, can eat into the enamel and make teeth more susceptible to cavities. There is a way around this, however. For citrus juices, lemonade, or undiluted lemon juice, you can sip it through a straw so that it reaches your throat and bypasses your teeth. Or, *immediately* after taking any of these enamel weakeners, rinse your mouth so that they do not remain on your teeth. Many people drink the juice of half a lemon in hot water first thing in the morning. This should not cause enamel erosion providing your mouth is promptly and thoroughly rinsed afterward with clear water.

Q. I am confused about the use of lemon. There are conflicting reports about its use. Should it be mixed with other foods? Even though acid, does it have an alkaline reaction in the stomach? Is it true that it is heavily sprayed and the skin is contaminated with pesticides?

Also, is brewer's yeast a complete source of vitamin B? How do the debittered, the bitter, the powder and the flakes compare?—A.W., Port Alberni, Canada

A. All non-organically raised citrus fruit is sprayed. Unless you have plenty of hydrochloric acid, cooked pineapple, tomatoes, sweet milk and citrus fruit can make you over-alkaline.

Brewer's, or nutritional yeast, is a powerhouse! It not only contains all of the B vitamins, but 16 amino acids (protein) and 15 minerals as well. Read your labels to determine if it is debittered for better flavor. Flakes are usually considered better in flavor by some people, although it requires more of them than the powder to provide the same amount of nutrients.

Q. I have been trying for a long time to obtain information about the nutritional value of fresh coconut juice. A friend highly recommends the drink but I have read that coconut oil is a saturated fat and should not be used in large quantites. I would like your opinion.—H.K., Los Angeles, California

A. According to *Composition and Facts About Foods* by Ford Heritage, the coconut contains calcium, some sodium, large amounts of magnesium and still larger amounts of potassium, plus iron, phosphorus, vitamins B-1, B-2, and niacin, as well as protein.

Gordon Fraser reports that in Thailand, Hawaii, and Mexico, the jelly of the immature green coconut, which is available there and made into a drink and kept iced, is both delicious and nutritious. He believes that this immature coconut is far superior to the hard meat of the mature coconut which is shipped to this country. However, he has an excellent solution for using even the hard meat of this type of coconut, usually quite indigestible, to good advantage. His recipe for a delight-ful and nutritious drink: 1 coconut to 10 carrots. Feed one piece of the coconut meat into a juicer, then 1 piece of carrot, until all is used. He says that the unsaturated fat is diluted with the carrot. Even so, he warns to use no more than 3 oz. of this juice at a time because it is a powerhouse, and any extra amount will place a burden on the liver (with the fat content) and on the pancreas (with the sugar content). Used in this way, he considers it a "heavenly drink."

Q. i read recently that coffee beans contain about 14 percent ether extract, which, due to its solubility, might result in one cupful of ether extract in every nine to 10 cups of coffee. The writer said that since this ether extract is taken into the stomach, it is much more dangerous than ether which is used in the hospitals, which only goes into the lungs. Is it true that coffee contains ether extract?—I.T., Brooklyn, New York

A. I called Frank Lachle, the chemical engineer, an expert on extractions of oils. Coffee contains some oils, but Frank Lachle said that the information is false. *Your coffee does not contain ether extract!* According to Webster's dictionary, ether extract consists chiefly of fats and fatty acids. It is not the same as ether gas used for anesthetics. In the laboratory, the chemist uses ether extract, a solvent, also known as petrolic ether, to determine the amount of oil solubles in any oily product. The amount used in this test is in only a small *sample*—perhaps three or four grams, *not* the entire product! Therefore, since not the whole product, or all the coffee beans, but only a few of them are tested and are probably thrown away after they are tested, there is no ether extract in the remaining coffee.

Q. The first thing I take in the morning is a beverage which includes one rounded teaspoon of dried mint tea, juice of half a lemon from my own tree, the lemon peel cut fine, and a cup and one-half of boiling water. I let this steep for 10 to 20 minutes, strain, and add honey. Do I get any appreciable amount of bioflavonoids from the peel, or am I merely wasting my time cutting it?—H.R., Piedmont, California

A. I have no analysis of lemon peel, but while there

are approximately 100 mgs. of vitamin C in a glass of orange juice, there are 1,000 mgs. of bioflavonoids in the white membrane of the fruit. However, in order to get this amount of bioflavonoids, it is undoubtedly necessary to eat the membrane (plus peel). You might put half a lemon, in whole form, into your blender for a few seconds and then add it to your tea. It will make a slightly chewy mixture, but at least you will be getting the entire benefit of the fruit, including the juice.

Q. What fruits contain glucose and what fruits contain fructose?—P.U., Tucson, Arizona

A. First, let's differentiate between glucose and fructose. Glucose is called *dextrose* and *grape sugar*. It is also the normal sugar present in the blood. In diabetes, the amount of glucose in the blood increases and very often spills over into the urine. Glucose occurs in fruits and vegetables. It is more than half the entire solid matter of honey and grapes.

Fructose is also called *levulose* and *fruit sugar*. It is present in sweet fruits together with glucose. It also occurs in starches and honey. It is sweeter than cane sugar (called sucrose) and is more easily assimilated. It, too, occurs in many vegetables.

No source of information I found was specific in separating the fruits in which fructose and glucose appear individually, since both appear together in grapes, cherries, bananas, etc.

## Sweets and Snacks

Q. I have read that there is no such thing as raw sugar, that it is white sugar with some of the molasses poured back into it. I have also read that the sugar cane is sprayed with very harmful insecticides and the fields are burned before harvesting, making anything derived from this process harmful. Is this true?—D.S., Houston, Texas

A. I asked Betty Morales for help with this question. Not only does she, with John T. Clark, own Organicville in Los Angeles, but the Sun Circle Ranch as well, which provides organic food now shipped all over the United States. Betty and John have traveled the world over (they are now in Hunza land) and have witnessed food and health conditions first-hand, rather than depending on second-hand information. Betty agrees that there is no such thing as raw sugar; sugar cane juice is extracted and boiled before being crystalized into sugar. She also agrees that the process of spraying and burning is true and that no sugar product is organically grown. She, as do others, believes that any refined sugar is not recommended nutritionally. However, some of the so-called "raw sugars" are slightly more nutritious than others. Here is Betty's rating of refined "raw sugars."

1. Yellow D contains the most molasses (rich in nutrients), thus the most minerals and the most B vitamins of all the "raw sugars." This is proved by analysis, which has been published.

2. Golden C is next in value, not completely refined, and only slightly less nutritious than Yellow D.

3. Kleen-raw is merely white sugar with molasses added. Fred Rohe states that five percent molasses is added; for light brown sugar, 12 percent molasses is added; and 13 percent is added for dark brown sugar. Drop a spoonful into water and watch the molasses wash away from the white sugar.

No one seems to have the complete information about Demerara and Turbinado sugar. Betty Morales and Paul Keene, owner of the mail order health food company in Penns Creek, Pennsylvania (for those who do not have access to health stores), both believe that Turbinado is only a partially refined sugar. Demerara, formerly imported from Cuba, but no longer available in this country, is described by the processors as "raw sugar" before it is turned into crystal white sugar.

Fred Rohe, a health food distributor and store owner, refuses to sell any sugar at all. He recommends as nutritionally accepted substitutes, honey, molasses, carob syrup and molasses, unrefined sugar cane syrup and date sugar.

Q. I have a teen-ager who is addicted to chocolate in any form. I tell her it is not good for her, particularly for her skin. She is not convinced. Are there other disturbing side effects of chocolate?—M.M.B., Winston-Salem, North Carolina

A. Some dermatologists now believe chocolate does not affect teen-age skin. But Adelle Davis states that chocolate interferes with the body's use of calcium, which explains why she does not approve of chocolate milk, particularly used in schools as a regular beverage. I have witnessed one family who used chocolate in an otherwise good health drink. The entire family, parents and children, were nervous, edgy and irritable, all symptoms of calcium deficiency. When the chocolate was discontinued and the calcium stepped up, the symptoms tapered off.

There is now new evidence against chocolate. A physician studying 164 patients states that eating chocolate caused heart attacks and angina in many of them. (*American Journal of Clinical Nutrition*, Jan., 1970)

Buy some carob powder at the health store—it tastes quite similar to chocolate. Let your daughter make some brownies from the recipes included and substitute them for the chocolate she craves. She may want to experiment until she finds the combination of ingredients so that the carob brownies taste like the real thing. I use honey, pecans, vanilla, sometimes a dash of cinnamon or dried Sanka or coffee together with unbleached flour, eggs and carob powder. I do not use baking powder, since I like chewey brownies instead of fluffy ones. So turn your daughter loose in the kitchen to experiment. You may find the entire family asking her to make more.

Q. I adore chocolate but it produces migraine headaches and skin blemishes for me. Why is this? Is there some way around it?—Mrs. M.B., Kalamazoo, Michigan

A. I was told by two people who had a checkup at the Mayo Clinic that about 90% of the population is allergic to chocolate. You may be one of this 90%, which may account for your migraine—an allergic response in some people. Chocolate is high in fat, which is why dermatologists forbid it for teen-agers suffering from acne. It contains oxalic acid, and Adelle Davis states that it leaches calcium from the body. It does contain a few vitamins, but it is high in calories, as everybody knows.

I am constantly surprised that so few people know about carob, which tastes very much like chocolate and comes from a long bean which grows on a tree. It was known in Biblical times as St. John's Bread. It is obtainable in powder form, and it contains only 1.4 grams of fat per 100 grams, as compared to 32.3 for chocolate. It also contains 15 minerals, vitamin A, and the B vitamins: thiamin, riboflavin and niacin. It is available at all health stores. You may have to experiment with it to get the flavor which tastes most nearly like chocolate, but it can be done. I use it exclusively as a chocolate substitute.

Q. In the advertisements, even some athletic coaches recommend sugar to increase energy. After reading of the bad effects of sugar, we are trying to eliminate it in our family diet. However, overcoming a sweet tooth is not easy. Any suggestions?—F.O., Cambridge, Massachusetts

A. Honey may be your answer. A young woman who helps me occasionally with my housework is slow but thorough. She doesn't always finish all the chores by quitting time, and leaves feeling tired. The other day she breezed through her work, finishing ahead of time, and still had energy to spare. When I commented on her excellent job and swift work, she said: "Do you know why? I took three teaspoons of natural honey before I left home and I have felt more energetic ever since."

This is worth a try for anybody: men, women, children and athletes, unless they are diabetics or hypoglycemics (low blood sugar patients). If you are a hypoglycemic and feel tired or shaky an hour or so after taking honey, you may need to cut your honey down or out completely. If you are a diabetic ask your doctor if he will permit you to have tupelo honey, which is often used for diabetics.

Natural, organic, unrefined honey is widely available and contains more vitamins and minerals than the clarified, heated, "de luxe" brands.

Q. Has glycerin, U.S.P., been analyzed as to proteins, carbohydrates and fat? When it is in distilled water, used as a skin lotion, it has a sweet flavor. Could it be tolerated as a substitute for other sweetening flavors in carbohydrate-limited diets?—F.H., San Antonio, Texas

A. Glycerin was first obtained as a by-product from fats and oils in the manufacture of soaps and fatty acids. It also becomes a natural product as a result of certain kinds of fermentation, especially the alcoholic fermentation of sugar. Therefore, it exists in many fermented wines and liquors. (About 1/30 of the sugar of grape juice fermented into alcohol becomes converted into glycerin.) In some natural fatty acids, such as palm oil, it exists in the free state and can be separated by washing the oil with boiling water, which dissolves the glycerin but not the fatty substances.

Just prior to World War II, glycerin began to be synthesized from propylene (a by-product of petroleum). Up to that time the natural glycerin was used externally as a softening agent; and internally as a laxative, preservative and solvent, and sometimes as a sweetening agent in place of sugar. It is still used as a sweetener in confections, an emollient in cosmetics, and as an aid in keeping fabrics pliable. It is also used as an anti-freeze, in elastic glues, printing inks, liquid soaps, and of course in nitroglycerin or dynamite. It is a syrupy liquid with a warm, sweet taste, and because it absorbs moisture from the air, it can act as a skin moisturizer. I find no analysis of protein, fat or carbohydrate content, but since it is so sweet, it undoubtedly has a high carbohydrate content.

Long ago I obtained some natural glycerin from a nutritional physician. I do not know if any is obtainable today. Since most glycerin now on the market is synthetic, I, personally, would not wish to take it internally, at least not until more information is available. However, used for skin care in a lotion mixed with distilled water, or incorporated into a moisturizer cosmetic, it is considered helpful by some people. Others find that it can irritate their skin.

Q. I do not allow my children to eat foodless snacks, including potato chips which, I understand, have very little nourishment and are also deep fat fried, thus I consider them somewhat indigestible. How about popcorn? Is it nutritious?—(No Signature)

A. It is an excellent snack, and a whole grain. And it is certainly full of nutrition. One cupful of popped popcorn contains the following:
* Protein—12.7 grams (higher than fruits or vegetables).
* Fat—5.0 grams (considered low; potato chips have over 7 times as much fat).
* Calories—386 (less than the same amount of graham crackers or peanuts).
* Minerals—11 mgs. of calcium, 281 mgs. phosphorus, 240 mgs. potassium and 2.7 mgs. iron.
* Vitamins—moderate amounts of the B complex.

## Assorted Food Queries

### SATURATED OILS

Q. I am enclosing a clipping of a newspaper column written by a medical doctor who states that the process of heating any unsaturated oil to ordinary cooking temperatures turns it into a saturated fat. I have been so careful to use cold-pressed safflower and other vegetable oils for cooking. Now it turns out it is of no value when heated. Do you agree with that?—A.N., Oakland, California

A. This same question popped up when the woman who made the homemade nutritious bread was quoted in this column as saying that a so-called "expert" told her the same thing. I don't know how this rumor got started, but as I said before, according to Frank Lachle, the chemical engineer who was in the edible oil refining business for 20 years and now owns a health store, the statement is *false*. Mr. Lachle, whose information has proved trustworthy, states that heating merely changes the molecule in the oil, but *does not cause the oil to become saturated.* So, relax, everybody.

## NATURAL FOOD CAMPS

Q. Can you help us locate summer resident camps for boys and girls that will serve them only natural foods?—Mr. and Mrs. A.R., Apopka, Florida

A. I turned to Beatrice Trum Hunter, author of *The Natural Foods Cookbook,* for help with this question. She suggests writing to Dr. Clark, director of the former North Country School, whose premises are now used by a summer camp which continues with the organically raised foods, a feature of the late North Country School. Dr. Clark's address is Lake Placid, N.Y. 12946. You might also write Natural Food Associates, Atlanta, Texas 75551. They may know of other possibilities.

## MEATS

Q. I would appreciate any information you can give concerning the value of kosher meat from the health viewpoint as distinguished from the religious viewpoint. Is it worthwhile going to a little extra trouble to get kosher meat?—H.L.N., Oakland, California

A. In the book *Baldness, Is It Necessary?* by Katherine Pugh, the author states that kosher meat is superior because it has not been injected with hormones.

John N. S. White, former meat inspection veterinarian, U.S. Department of Agriculture, writes (National Health Federation *Bulletin,* January 1970) that stilbestrol, a female sex hormone, used for increasing weight gain in cattle, is recognized by the National Cancer Institute as a cancer-producing substance. For this reason, he recommends that "ALL forms of stilbestrol medication, either by injection or medication, should be discontinued." Dr. White tells of examining the carcass of a hormone treated steer "which had mammary glands as large as a cow's, and milk could be expressed easily from the teats." This animal had been sent to a meat packing house for processing.

Studies in Denmark, England, Israel and the United States show that some male workers in factories producing the artificial female sex hormones develop womanly type breasts, lose their beards and become impotent by merely breathing the tiny particles of the hormones. For this reason there is a law banning the use of these hormones in American meat, but the practice still continues illegally, according to Dr. White. He says, "There is a definite conflict of interest between the U.S. Department of Agriculture Meat Inspection Service and the cattle raising industry." Many farmers apparently still slyly use the sex hormones to increase the weight of the animal and the money in their pocket.

Kosher food, on the other hand, is rigidly supervised by a qualified inspector to assure, for religious purposes (which often turn out to be healthful practices), that no foreign substance is injected into or mixed with it. I double checked with Jewish authorities, who stated that no hormone injections are allowed. A kosher butcher added, "No shots; it's against our religion."

I did not get a clear answer, however, whether or not the kosher inspection could pinpoint animals which had been given *feed* which contained the sex hormones. After all, the inspection is motivated, not by health, but by religion. Kosher meat is also not avilable in many communities.

The safest solution is to buy *organically* raised meat, which not only bypasses hormone feed, medication, and injections, but insecticides and other chemical treatments, as well. Such meat, admittedly, is hard to get and more expensive. Health food stores often carry it in frozen form or can perhaps direct you to recommended sources of supply.

To get *any* kind of unadulterated food takes extra time, effort and money. But many people believe it pays for itself in the long run in lowered health costs, and is therefore well worth it.

Q. Are cooked clams safe to eat? I understand that raw clams and oysters may cause trouble.—J.H., Santa Ana, California

A. It is true that raw clams and oysters from contaminated waters, even where pollution is not suspected, have been found to cause hepatitis. Experts agree that for every reported case there are one to five unreported cases of hepatitis caused by eating this type of shellfish. Four physicians, writing in the *New England Journal of Medicine* (April, 1967), stated that the hazard is continual, not seasonal. And of 185 cases of hepatitis studied, at least 25 per cent had caught the disease from eating this type of shellfish. Of those affected, raw as well as steamed shellfish had been eaten. The physicians said that most steaming is insufficient to kill the hepatitis virus, but if the entire batch of clams (on the inside as well as the outside layer of the batch) is exposed to live steam for at least five minutes, the virus can be inactivated. Frying or other means of cooking is safe as long as it is thorough, the physicians stated.

## RAW FOODS

Q. My elderly sister eats only cooked foods because she claims that raw foods hurt her stomach. She will eat morning cereal, and for other meals, meat, potatoes and cooked vegetables, plus toasted white bread. I tell her she should eat raw salads but she is afraid they will hurt her stomach. What do you think?—M.O., Mesa, Arizona

A. Everyone needs raw foods, since they contain vitamins and minerals undamaged by heat, and enzymes which are considered the housecleaners of the body. But most people also eat some cooked food such as corn, potatoes and meat. Actually, a study has revealed that cooked carrots help the body to assimilate more vitamin A than raw carrots. Many health-minded doctors and nutritionists, however, recommend that at least 50% of the diet should be raw if you wish to maintain good health. The raw foods should be organic, if possible (raised with no sprays or chemicals).

In elderly people, poor teeth may make it difficult to chew raw foods thoroughly. If one can chew them until they become almost liquid, they should be easier on the digestion. However, if teeth are poor, or there are dentures, the answer is a juicer. All raw fruits and vegetables can then be put in delicious juice form and provide the body with the necessary and beneficial nutrients found in raw foods.

## EDIBLE PLANTS

Q. I have been reading some books on eating wild plants. It is fascinating reading but I wonder if experimentation is safe for the non-expert? Like mushrooms, for instance. I couldn't tell the difference between a safe and a poisonous species.—M.M., Richmond, Virginia

A. You are so right. You should not eat the roots, fruits, flowers or stems of any plant, even a familiar one, until you are *sure* it is safe. Carol Bacon, the wife of a pharmacist and director of the San Francisco area Poison Prevention Committee, lists some examples:

*Poinsettia*—Leaves, stem and flower can cause vomiting, temporary blindness, possibly delirium.

*Rhubarb*—Stalk is edible; leaf can cause severe abdominal cramps or, in large amounts, coma and death.

*Potato*—Green sprouts on the edible portion, shoots, leaves and stem can cause mental confusion, cardiac depression, sometimes death.

*Rhododendron*—Entire plant is toxic, causing muscle paralysis, convulsions, then death, 3 to 14 hours after fatal dose has been ingested.

*Cherry Tree*—Twigs, leaves, bark and fruit stones form cyanide in body.

Other poisonous plants are foxglove, buttercup, iris, lily-of-the-valley, sweet pea, wisteria and oleander. Children have died from nibbling the oleander blossoms, leaves and twigs. Contact with the bush may cause skin irritation.

Beans of castor oil plant are also dangerous. Eating even two beans has proved fatal.

# VITAMINS AND SUPPLEMENTS

## VITAMIN A

Q. A fellow on TV said the other day that over 25,000 units of vitamin A per day would cause cancer of the lungs. Is this right?— C.L.W., Marienville, Pennsylvania

A. It would be interesting to know if the statement of this "fellow" was his own opinion or the result of a scientific study. It is true that vitamin A and vitamin D are the two vitamins which, used in overdoses for *some* people, can produce toxicity. If this occurs, and the vitamin is stopped, the symptoms disappear. The reaction seems to be an individual matter, however. Adelle Davis, in her book, *Let's Get Well,* says, "Physicians have given 150,000 to 300,000 units of vitamin A daily for varying periods with no signs of toxicity, and no fatalities have ever been reported."

She adds, "Massive amounts of vitamin A or carotene have stopped the growth of spontaneous cancers in mice. When 300,000 units of vitamin A and 1,000 milligrams of vitamin C were given daily for three to six months to 218 cases [in humans] of inoperable cancer, the malignancies regressed in size or remained stationary."

Miss Davis' statements are not her own opinions, but the results of scientific studies which she documents in her book under the heading of medical references.

## VITAMIN E

Q. Recently in my area I heard an FDA telephone "educational message" in which a person calls a number and is given a three-minute message on various subjects. This one was on vitamin E and the listener was told that we really do not need to take vitamin E; that we get enough in our food. If we still want to take it, we were told, we should take it in the form of wheat germ, or if we insist on a supplement, we should not take more than the recommended daily allowance, which is 30 I.U. daily, unless supervised by a physician. What is your opinion of this information?—B.F., Mill Valley, California

A. I have written about vitamin E in the nutrition course which has already appeared in *Let's LIVE,* quoting the findings of many experts on the subject. I still believe that anyone who wishes to take vitamin E should read the informative book, *Vitamin E for Ailing and Healthy Hearts,* by Wilfred E. Shute, M.D. (published by Pyramid Publications, and available through health or book stores in hardback only). This book provides reliable information from a physician, who, with his brother, Dr. Evan Shute, has rehabilitated more than 30,000 cases of heart ailments with the correct dosages of vitamin E.

A recent study in Great Britain found that after reduction of freshness in foods through storage, as well as loss through cooking, there often is not enough of a nutrient left in the food to supply even the *minimum* daily requirement. The researchers found that in three-quarters of the diets studied, the average food supplied less than five I.U.'s of vitamin E daily. Furthermore, these researchers suspect that many people may take vitamin E without assimilating it properly.

Because our food is so highly refined and vitamin E is removed from grains, along with the precious wheat germ because it is perishable and has a short shelf life, the Doctors Shute advocate much higher potencies of vitamin E than the recommended daily allowances. I suggest you read the Shute book.

Q. I noticed in your review of Dr. Shute's book, *Vitamin E for Ailing and Healthy Hearts,* that estrogen destroys vitamin E if taken at the same time. I was really dismayed to learn this since I had been taking vitamin E and estrogen together for 9 months. I am ensuring that this does not happen in the future! This raises another question: does estrogen destroy other vitamins? Also, what is organic iron? And what are the merits of safflower oil?—Mrs. J.D.I., Montreal, Canada

A. To my knowledge, estrogen does not destroy other vitamins. However, there are some other antagonists to other vitamins. There is an enzyme in raw clams and oysters which destroys vitamin B1 (thiamin). Sulfa drugs destroy vitamin B2 in the body. Penicillin and chloromycetin have been reported as destroying nicotinic acid in the system. (Nicotinic acid is a B vitamin.) *Any* drug (including tranquilizers, sleeping pills and aspirin) will destroy vitamin C. Mineral oil destroys all of the fat soluble vitamins (A, D, E, K). Bleaching agents, used to bleach white flour, destroys vitamin E, and dicoumerol, a blood-thinning drug, as well as the sulfa drugs, destroy vitamin K needed for normal blood clotting.

Other vitamin antagonists include arsenic, lead, bismuth, and mercury, if used in drugs, or some of them in large amounts in chemical fertilizers on foods. Sulfuring of foods also destroys vitamins, and the nitrates and nitrites deposited in vegetables by chemical fertilizers, or added to most frankfurters and cold processed meats as well as baby foods, destroy vitamin A. Rancid fat in the diet causes a loss of vitamins A and E. High amounts of chlorine in the water react against vitamins in the digestive tract; vitamin E is the greatest target. And chemical vapors in the polluted air around factories destroy vitamins A, B, C, and K in our bodies.

The solution to this alarming problem of vitamin losses is one reason you subscribe to *Let's LIVE:* to learn how to avoid processed food and how to fortify your diet with the proper vitamins to make up for the loss.

Organic iron is derived from living sources, usually of food and animal origin.

Safflower oil is a highly polyunsaturated oil. This means it has a high solubility factor and dissolves more fat in the body and blood stream than some other oils. It is also easier to digest, but by the same token, spoils more easily. To prevent oxidization (rancidity) in the body by a highly polyunsaturated oil, more vitamin E is necessary. Preventing rancidity in the bottle is helped by buying it in small amounts, and after unsealing, keeping it in the refrigerator.

## MEGA VITAMINS

Q. I am a heartbroken mother. My son, age 21, is now in a state hospital and has been in and out of mental hospitals for the past four years. Nothing yet has alleviated his hostility and aggressiveness. My son used to be an A student, had high hopes for his future, but now knows only hopelessness and suppressed rage.

I have read of the mega-vitamin therapy for the treatment of mental disease. I refer specifically to Doctors Hoffer and Osmund and Linus Pauling's theory that mental illness can be due to a chemical imbalance which can be reversed by the intake of large amounts of vitamin B-3 (niacin), C, and glutamic acid. When I mention this mega-vitamin therapy to the doctors, I feel both their pity and amusement. As one doctor put it, I am clutching at a straw. I need proof for these doctors that this theory does work. Please help me.—Mrs. F.W., Los Angeles, California

A. The word "mega" is a word element meaning "great amount." A megaphone, for example, greatly magnifies sound. Thus, mega-vitamin therapy merely means large amounts of the vitamins mentioned.

Linus Pauling, the Nobel prize winner, has recommended massive doses of vitamin C for mental illness on the basis of a successful study done in Texas.

Abram Hoffer, M.D., Ph.D., and Humphrey Osmond, M.R.C.S., D.P.M., have written a book, *How to Live with Schizophrenia* (University Books, New Hyde Park, New York, 1966), after their successful use of massive doses of niacin, a B vitamin which they call vitamin B-3. Victims of this mental disturbance begin to suffer from delusions and lose touch with the world. Some patients become mute and withdrawn. Others feel persecuted. Still others become extravagant and silly. According to Dr. Hoffer, the sooner the disease, which usually strikes persons between the late teens and the age of 30, is caught, the easier it is to cure. In early stages the use of niacin and vitamin C may be enough to help the patient. In more complicated cases the treatment is accompanied by the use of antidepressants, tranquilizers and psychotherapy.

Dr. Hoffer says that though there is not a single

published paper attacking the vitamin treatment, there is a "current myth" among doctors that the treatment is not successful. "I can assure you," he adds, "that every doctor who has not tried it is against it."

There are two facts about niacin which, I believe, should be known. Although it is true that the Hoffer-Osmond method has worked in many, many cases, it is my opinion that the vitamin therapy should not be restricted to these vitamins alone. Reports indicate that the administration of a single B vitamin without benefit of the other companion B vitamins naturally occurring in the vitamin B complex has led to side effects. For example, Arthur U. Rivin, M.D., found that 3 to 6 grams of synthetic niacin given to a 23-year-old man for reducing his cholesterol resulted in jaundice. There are other cases of different side effects. Another fact often not told a patient by a doctor who prescribes niacin for various other ailments is that this vitamin usually causes an intense flush. The person turns beet red, itches and feels hot. Although the reaction is extremely frightening to one who is not prepared for it, it lasts only about 20 minutes and is harmless. It merely speeds up circulation to a high degree to different parts of the body. Niacinamide is the same vitamin, minus the flushing activity. It is niacin, however, which is used by Doctors Hoffer and Osmund.

Roger J. Williams, Ph.D., head of the Department of Chemistry at University of Texas and a discoverer of pantothenic acid, one of the B vitamins, reported a dramatic case in which niacin was given to a mentally disturbed woman who thought her neighbors were conspiring to kill her. Within 48 hours after being given niacin, her attitude became normal. Dr. Williams, in commenting on niacin deficiency, which is usually associated with pellagra (a nutritional deficiency disease), says, "Many have received similar benefits and there is no doubt that nutritional supplementation in these cases is capable of revolutionizing one's thinking and acting."

I have personally observed a normally intelligent

young married woman with five children who became mentally disturbed. Psychotherapy and a short term of hospitalization by a psychiatrist did not permanently relieve her condition. A nutritional analysis revealed that she herself was forgetting to follow good nutritional principles (which she understood) in favor of keeping up with the needs of her family. At a nutritionist's suggestion she began taking niacin on her own, as she tapered off the tranquilizer given her by her doctor (using it only for emergencies). She also took vitamin C, the *full* B complex in the form of brewer's yeast, liver and a natural vitamin B syrup. To the joy of her family and friends, she is a normal, well person today.

One other possible cause of mental illness is low blood sugar (hypoglycemia). I also wonder if drugs, or alcoholism, or both, which reduce a person's judgment and his appetite for proper nutritional substances, might be a factor in some cases of mental illness.

My suggestion is to purchase a copy of the Hoffer-Osmund book, written by two respectable M.D.'s about their use of the mega-vitamin therapy for a 15-year period, and loan it to your doctors to read. Perhaps after they have read it, you could ask them to try the therapy as a test case on your son. When he is home again, perhaps you could initiate a complete nutritional program to finish the job.

## WHEAT GERM

Q. Can the germ of the wheat be extracted at home to make fresh wheat germ? If so, is there any literature describing this process?—J.G.S., Ottawa, Canada

A. I am sorry to say that I know of no literature on this subject of home extraction of wheat germ. It is usually done by heavy, expensive rolling equipment in large commercial flour mills.

You are very wise in wishing to acquire fresh wheat germ, since it is so delicate that it soon begins to oxidize because of the oil content. This is why fresh wheat germ should be refrigerated both in health stores as well as in homes, and wheat germ oil should be refrigerated the minute it is opened and comes in contact with the air.

There are several alternatives. Wheat germ oil can be purchased in air-tight capsules. If you cannot find fresh wheat germ, kept under refrigeration, then the vacuum-packed, usually lightly toasted and really more palatable, is usually available at health stores. Best of all, however, is to get either fresh-ground whole grain flour at the mill, or by grinding your own wheat, you get the benefits of the whole grain, including the germ.

There are some small electric grinders which can grind a few wheat berries at a time, which might suffice for a daily serving of fresh-ground cereal, eaten raw, if you wish. Or perhaps you could buy with some other families a heavy duty home mill to grind your own flour for making bread. The flavor of this fresh ground flour in home-made bread is incomparable.

The wheat germ, again, remains sealed in each wheat berry and thus is protected against the air until it is ground. By using the entire product of wheat and germ, you receive the advantages of the B vitamins as well as vitamin E which occurs in the germ. There are a *few* health stores which will grind the flour before your eyes. It should be used promptly, so buy only enough for your immediate needs.

## BREWER'S YEAST

Q. Is brewer's yeast fattening?—A.M., Cambridge, Massachusetts

A. No. There are 1400 calories in an entire pound, or only 80 calories in one tablespoon, or in 90 tablets. Brewer's yeast is high in protein, vitamins and minerals, and thus is considered an almost complete reducing food.

However, there is one caution to observe: It is extremely high in phosphorus. Phosphorus and calcium are as closely related as twins, and when phosphorus is washed out of the body it tends to take the calcium with it, leading to nervousness or jitters.

This does not apply just to yeast, but to many proteins. It is easily remedied. People on a high protein diet, or those taking a large amount of brewer's yeast daily, need only to step up their calcium intake. This requirement could be satisfied by milk in some form (including yogurt, buttermilk or skim milk powder). Or you can add ¼ cup of calcium lactate powder or ½ cup of calcium gluconate to each pound of brewer's yeast and mix well. I swish mine around in a large paper sack before storing it in a smaller container. Then it is always ready to use. I add a tablespoon or more of the mixture to juice whenever I need a pick-up.

Q. I have read in several nutrition books that it takes 90 tablets of brewer's yeast to equal one tablespoon of powdered yeast. Isn't this a mistake?—F.R., Portland, Oregon

A. I have quoted Adelle Davis in my own books as making this statement. However, new yeasts are being bred and potencies change. Betty Morales and John T. Clark, of Eden Ranch (Organicville) in Los Angeles, give a more recent and perhaps more realistic equivalent in their *Organic Consumer Report* (Aug. 17, 1971). They state, "It takes 24 yeast tablets to equal one level tablespoon of brewer's yeast."

## CALCIUM . . .

Q. What kind of calcium is best?—E.L.M., Medford, Oregon

A. This is a hard question to answer because different calciums apparently are utilized differently by different people. I have seen tests conducted in which six varieties of calcium were tested for one individual. Five of them did not do the job. The sixth did. Also different types of calcium are apparently needed for different functions in the body. For example, bone meal seems to help particularly in strengthening teeth and bones and in more rapid healing following fractures. In other words, bone is helped by bone. Other forms of calcium may be necessary for tissues and muscles (the heart is a muscle and needs calcium). Some calciums are more soluble than others and are more quickly taken up by the body. They include calcium lactate, calcium glyconate and calcium levulinate. The less soluble forms of calcium include bone meal, dolomite and dicalcium phosphate. Unless the body produces enough HCL (digestive acid) the less soluble calciums may not be dissolved and thus made useful for the body. I have recently discovered a phosphorus-free calcium in health stores which includes all in one product, various kinds of calcium including that from oyster shells. It also contains magnesium and some HCL to help calcium digestion. Since this product does not yet contain bone meal, I add it on the side, to be sure I get all the varieties I need.

## . . . AND MAGNESIUM

Q. My customers (I own a health food store) and I are concerned about two things. We have read that magnesium, being an antacid, should not be taken along with calcium since calcium needs an acid medium for assimilation. Yet there are preparations which contain both. How can these both be assimilated or utilized if they are so opposite? Since so many people lack hydrochloric acid, how do they use any calcium and/or magnesium?

The other question is about water. Are those of us who are using distilled water and boiling our water for an hour doing right? Why does distilled water leach out minerals? Another writer who has published a book about water does not say anything about distilled water leaching minerals out of the body.—A Health Store Owner, Arkansas

A. Please remember that I am a reporter only. When a technical question comes in, like "Dear Abby," I call upon experts who specialize in the subject. In the case of magnesium, calcium and its assimilation, I received this information from experts who work with and constantly test the effects of these minerals:

There is one magnesium, magnesium gluconate, which is *not* an antacid. It can be combined with calcium without disturbing the acid medium needed for calcium utilization. However, it contains a very low percentage of magnesium.

Because research shows that most Americans are deficient in magnesium and need a higher potency than that supplied by magnesium gluconate, other types of magnesium are generally used. Since they *are* antacids, if they are taken between meals they do not disturb the acid medium needed at meal times for the proper digestion of calcium (also protein and iron). However, if a product is taken which combines magnesium and calcium, some people may need hydrochloric acid. (What kind and how much to take is explained by a doctor in my book, *Secrets of Health and Beauty*.) At least one company adds hydrochloric acid to a calcium-magnesium combination. This product is one solution to the problem. Remember that people differ. One frantic mother wrote me that she could not give her children magnesium between meals because they were at school. Most children have a plentiful supply of stomach acid, as some adults do. I find a convenient time to take magnesium is just before bedtime. Several people, who were puzzled because symptoms of calcium shortage continued in spite of their generous intake of a calcium/magnesium product, wrote me that they noted improvement when they took the minerals separately—calcium with meals and magnesium between meals. Each person must experiment to learn his own pattern, however.

Now about water. I am literally flooded with questions from people who are understandably concerned about the problem of good drinking water. In addition to your questions, others ask how to get minerals if one drinks distilled water; and how water is de-ionized. Again, I went to experts including chemists and physicians. So these answers are a composite of what a group of experts told me.

First, let's look at the organic vs. the inorganic minerals in water. Hard water contains more minerals than soft water. World-wide research reveals that hard water areas show the least amount of heart trouble; soft water areas show the greatest amount of heart disturbance in the population. Both inorganic and organic minerals are needed by the body. This is proved in research done in connection with the Schuessler Cell Salts. On autopsy, the inorganic minerals are found in the ashes of a healthy body. If there is a deficiency of any of these minerals, organic or inorganic, health becomes disturbed. When they are resupplied and utilized, health improvement has been noted. Hard water contains more of these minerals. Sea water contains all of them. Please notice that I have said that if these minerals are supplied and *utilized*, health responds accordingly. There are many investigators who believe that arthritis is one example in which there is insufficient calcium intake or if there is enough calcium taken, because of insufficient acid, the calcium is not utilized and it piles up in unwanted places. Dr. Jarvis, in his book on Vermont Folk Medicine, likens it to the deposits on the inside of a tea kettle; if an apple cider vinegar solution is put in the tea kettle, the mineral deposits which had hardened on the surface are dissolved, leaving a clean surface. He reported that Vermonters used apple cider vinegar to keep minerals in solution in their bodies and those of their farm animals so they would not pile up in the joints or the heart or the tissues. Other therapists use hydrochloric acid for stomach acid deficiency. Thus minerals *and* acid are needed for correct utilization. If there is a deficiency of either, trouble may result.

Why does distilled water leach minerals out of the body? Because distilled water has had the minerals removed. In the body, there must be minerals for health since it has already been stated that minerals make up part of the body composition and must be constantly renewed. There must be a balance of all minerals in the body at all times for optimum health. If a mineral-free liquid such as distilled water is taken into the body, an exchange takes place through the body membranes. In a laboratory, if you stretch a membrane between two bodies of water, one salt, the other fresh, in due time, *both* bodies of water will become salty. If you stretch a membrane between one body of colored water and another uncolored body of water, in due time both will be colored. The exchange takes place in the same way through the body membranes. Thus if you put a mineral-free liquid into the body, the liquid (distilled water) will draw the minerals from the blood through the intestinal membrane and wash them out of the body.

So if you drink distilled water, minerals should be taken in it or with it to prevent this exchange, in order to compensate for the loss of minerals from the water. That is why many people who use distilled water add 8 tablespoons of filtered sea water (filtered to remove possible contaminants) to one gallon of distilled water.

Dr. Nittler gives another suggestion: To each 8-oz. glass of distilled water, add one-fourth teaspoon of sea salt or sea water (presumably contains all minerals) and 2 teaspoons of apple cider vinegar.

Ionizing water is another method of removing minerals from water. One example is that of a water softener. By running the hard water through salt, the other minerals are attracted away from the water and drawn off. This is why many who feel they must have soft water for laundry and dishwashing purposes do not have the cold water—used for beverages—attached to the water softener. They do not want to lose valuable minerals.

I am at a loss to understand why you boil your water an hour. Boiling removes chlorine. A few minutes will do the trick since, if you leave chlorinated water exposed to the air, it evaporates in a short time without boiling.

## CELL SALTS

Q. You mentioned that one of the cell salts is named calcium fluorica. I am interested in learning the difference, if any, between this product and fluoride which is used in drinking water.— G.D.McK., Columbus, Ohio

A. The fluoride which is added to drinking water is *sodium* fluoride, apparently considered toxic, as it accumulates in the system, according to anti-fluoridation investigators. The ingredient in the cell salt is quite different. It is *calcium* fluoride, also known as fluoride of lime. You can read about its values in books on Dr. Schuessler's cell salts, some of which I listed at the end of the article on cell salts. (This article appeared in the February 1970 issue of *Let's LIVE*.)

Q. Your recent article on cell salts is very interesting but I understand they are inorganic. A writer about water says that only the living plant has the power to extract inorganic minerals from the earth; no human can extract nourishment from inorganic minerals nor can the human body (according to this writer) handle the inorganic minerals. Since all 12 cell salts are inorganic minerals, this is very confusing to me. Can you clarify?—J.D., Rexdale, Ontario, Canada

A. In order to answer your question I checked with (1) a nutritional physician, (2) a nationally known chemist and biochemist (a Ph.D. and a specialist on minerals), and (3) an expert on cell salts who has witnessed their successful results on thousands of people for the 35 years he has spent in this field. All of these experts state that it is simply not true that the human body cannot assimilate or use inorganic minerals. (Organic minerals are those elements derived from animal or vegetable tissues; inorganic minerals come from soil or rocks. Many of the minerals are found in both sources.)

The nutritional physician said that one example is salt: during heart weakness he gives patients under his treatment a small amount of salt in a glass of water to sip and it revives the patient within minutes. The doctor stated that if he himself is working hard out of doors, is sweating profusely, he drinks a salt solution (he uses a teaspoon of sea salt to a glass of water) and this is taken in by the body immediately to provide energy. *Salt is an inorganic mineral.*

The biochemist specialist on minerals said that there is isotope proof that the body uses inorganic minerals. Isotopes mean that radioactive tracers are added to an element fed the body so that it can be seen by a special machine where it goes in the body. Different inorganic minerals go to various parts of the body. All scientists agree that *the body is made of inorganic minerals,* including a textbook on biochemistry (by Harrow and Mazur, 7th edition, published by W. B. Saunders Co., Philadelphia and London, 1958). This textbook states: "The common inorganic elements found in living tissues include calcium, magnesium, sodium, potassium, sulfur, phosphorus, chlorine, iron and iodine. The spectroscope has revealed traces of many other elements. . . . Many enzymes require small quantities of inorganic elements for their activity." (An enzyme is a catalyst, of organic nature, to help the body in its assimilation and thus establish equilibrium.)

J. B. Chapman, M.D., says: "The human body is composed of two kinds of matter, organic and inorganic . . . indeed the organic could not perform its proper function without the inorganic." Dr. Chapman adds, "The 12 inorganic (mineral) salts are all essential to the proper growth and development of every part of the system. . . . The inorganic substances in the blood and tissues are sufficient to heal all diseases which are curable at all . . . by replacing these lacking elements, an equilibrium will again be restored and the organism may return to its normal condition."

According to his book, *Biochemistry,* one-twentieth of the human body is composed of inorganic minerals and if there is a deficiency of any of them the balance of the body will be upset and health problems will follow the deficiencies.

It is indeed true that the human body does not *always* assimilate some of these inorganic minerals efficiently. If there is a shortage of hydrochloric acid in the stomach, for example, calcium or iron cannot be properly assimilated. In the case of calcium, it may pile up in unwanted places in the body instead of being dissolved by the digestive acid so that it can be used properly. This is the advantage of the 12 cell salts. The particles of these 12 inorganic minerals (all found in body ash) are reduced to such infinitesimal sizes that they are easily assimilated by the body cells and make "proper union with organic matter which they control," a method as closely similar to nature's method as possible.

The cell salt expert reminded me that these cell salts have been used with success all over the world for at least 100 years, although the medical profession frowns on them because they are homeopathic in nature instead of being drugs. As to inorganic minerals in the water, it is not the fault of the minerals but what the body does with them! A normal functioning body, with sufficient digestive acid, will dissolve and use them, rather than let them accumulate, and cause any possible trouble. Adding apple cider vinegar to your water or hydrochloric acid to your diet will solve the problem of lack of assimilation. Unless your water is fluoridated, or contaminated with detergents, relax and drink it up.

Q. After reading a book on drinking water, my husband insists on drinking distilled water. All it has done for him is to give him a sore knee, a sore elbow and terrific pains between the shoulder blades. When we went on our vacation we used only well water, and he never had a pain all the time we were gone. Still I cannot convince him that he needs water which contains all the minerals rather than water which has had them removed. I have also read that more heart attacks occur where the water is soft (low in minerals) than where it is hard (high in minerals). Could you tell me where I can get the cell salts in combination which contain the 12 different minerals so that he can take them with his distilled water? I love my husband too much to have him become a candidate for a heart attack.—Mrs. C.W., Tampa, Florida

A. Most homeopathic pharmacies carry the individual cell salts as well as the all-in-one combination I have mentioned.

# WATER

Q. Is it true that everyone should drink eight glasses of water daily?—D.F., San Francisco, California

A. Apparently this is an individual problem, influenced by many factors. According to Milton E. Rubini, M.D., Editor-in-Chief of the *American Journal of Clinical Nutrition* (July, 1970, p. 863), the desire and need for intake of water is based upon thirst of an individual. Thirst can be caused by a variety of factors: loss of blood (as anyone who has given a blood donation may have noticed); dryness of mouth and throat; physiological factors in disease (such as diabetes); as well as psychological influences.

Foods which cause thirst include chocolate as well as salty foods, including ham, anchovies and pretzels, as well as foods prepared or served with generous amounts of soy sauce (which may account for Orientals' desire for large amounts of tea with their meals).

According to Dr. Rubini, there is a great difference in various species of animals in their need for water. A man who works in the desert learns that at the end of the day his horse will drink the exact amount of water it has lost. On the other hand, a camel drinks only 50 per cent of its water deficit at the end of the day, gradually acquiring the rest while eating. States Dr. Rubini, "Man is more like a camel than a horse." He tells of troop commanders who tried to train men to require less water, with complete failure. It became clear during these attempts that each man has a rigid requirement for water based upon his own needs and this requirement cannot be changed at the insistence of a troop commander, or anyone else.

This, then, may explain the advice by some who

counsel, instead of the old rule of thumb, "Drink 8 glasses of water a day," a rule that applies better to the needs of each individual: drink water whenever you are thirsty.

**Q. Does boiling water for five minutes eliminate the minerals and some of the chlorine?—J.W.K.**

A. Boiling water removes all of the chlorine and none of the minerals. Chlorine will also evaporate if you leave a container of water uncovered overnight. In either case, the water can be refrigerated after chlorine removal.

## HARD VS. SOFT WATER

**Q. No. 1: We have recently moved to the Chicago area where, for the first time, we have a water softener. We have been using bottled spring water for beverages, tea, soup, etc., but it is becoming too expensive for a family of four. Which is really better for beverages, hard water or soft?—D.S.Z., Geneva, Illinois**
**Q. No. 2: After drinking chemical-laden city water, I experience a severe burning in the left shoulder, which doctors believe is an acid condition. For this reason I have been drinking distilled water for several years. Am I on the right track?—L.K.A., Kansas City, Missouri**

A. This is becoming a dilemma for many people: safe drinking water. It is true that buying bottled spring water is one solution, providing the bottled water is reliable and you can afford it. One bottling company on the West Coast recently discontinued their bottled spring water because it was found to contain detergents and other contaminants. They substituted distilled water to which they add minerals, and gave it a different name which sounds like spring water, but really isn't. So read your labels to be sure what you are getting.

*Consumer Bulletin,* March 1963, stated, "Dr. Henry A. Schroeder, Associate Professor of Clinical Physiology, Dartmouth Medical School, reported in 1960 that he had found that fewer people died from heart disease in places where water was relatively hard. The number of deaths was greater where soft water was consumed by the population. This finding was found valid both for the U.S. and England."

Soft water, softened water and distilled water do not contain the minerals found in hard water. One study showed that rabbits drinking distilled water had more hardening of the arteries than those drinking hard water. (*Archives of Pathology,* Vol. 73—No. 5, 1962)

Water softened by a home softener or a community water softener is higher in sodium (salt) content, since the softening process exchanges sodium for calcium and magnesium. Even some wells and rivers may be high in sodium. And of course chlorine is another chemical to reckon with, to say nothing of fluorine. Joseph M. Price, M.D., in a study of chickens, found that chlorine-treated water can cause heart attacks and strokes. Of course, the hazards of adding fluorine to drinking water are well documented, though still not accepted by some people.

This all adds up to a conclusion which reminds us of the old saying, "Water, water, everywhere and not a drop to drink." So what can you do?

If chlorine is your only problem, the solution is easy. It disappears on boiling and the water can then be refrigerated to use for beverages.

The next easiest problem to solve is a home water softener. Disconnect it from the cold water, but leave it connected to the hot water for bathing, dishes and laundry.

For fluorine, and other community-added chemicals, getting real bottled spring water, or distilling your own and adding valuable minerals removed by the distillation process may be your answer. Or you can add minerals to your diet in supplement form. To make sure I get enough, I take a mineral supplement, add the tablet to my distilled water, in addition to a teaspoon of purified sea water obtained in health stores. The result, after refrigeration, is a delightful, fresh-tasting water. Expensive to procure safe drinking water? Yes. But cheaper in the long run than poor health.

Q. I have had several arguments with people who drink distilled water. They insist that it is free from impurities, therefore safe.

Do you have any medical documentation to the contrary I can use to convince them?—B.W., Columbus, Ohio

A. It is quite true that distilled water is free of impurities, but by the same token it has also had minerals removed at the same time impurities were removed. A recent study in Canada revealed that in three territories where water was soft (containing few minerals) intermediate (containing more minerals) and hard water (high mineral content) the areas with soft water reported more sudden deaths from heart disease and more heart disease cases. There were less heart disturbances in the intermediate areas and least in the hard water locations. The documentation for this: *New England Journal of Medicine,* 1969, 280, 805-807).

This effect of soft water on hearts was confirmed in an English study. Also, bone calcium and magnesium were found lower in people living in soft water areas. (*Lancet* i 699-701)

Q. What minerals should be added to distilled water and in what amounts?—W.J.M., Sun City, California

A. Dr. Nittler and the late Dr. Royal Lee have stated that distilled water is a hypotonic solution which draws or leaches electrolytes from the body. In order to prevent this thievery from the body, the *hypotonic* solution of the distilled water can be changed to an *isotonic* solution by the addition of sea water, so that it will be balanced and not draw out the electrolytes and leach the minerals from the body. If you have a distiller which makes ½ gallon of distilled water nightly, add 4 teaspoonsful of safe, uncontaminated, filtered sea water from health stores. This makes the solution isotonic and imparts a good flavor. If you do not have a water distiller and do buy distilled water by the gallon, you would add 8 teaspoons of sea water.

In addition, step up the minerals in your diet to compensate for their removal from your original drinking water. (The sea water adds only traces of minerals.) Kelp products provide a complete spectrum of all minerals, known and unknown. As to amount, each person has different needs. Some people need more iodine than others. Since iodine occurs in kelp, is stimulating and helpful up to a point, too much might be overstimulating to some people. If you find yourself becoming slightly jittery, says Dr. Nittler, reduce your intake of kelp mineral tablets until this symptom vanishes.

Q. The bottled water I use is available from a large distributor for adjacent cities in the area. Formerly it came from natural springs. Now it is tap water, distilled, with minerals added and labeled so as to give the impression that it is still spring water. Can you tell me what these added minerals are and are we better off with this type of water than the original spring water?—S.P., San Anselmo, California

A. I called several experts and the heads of several bottled water plants, one being the largest distributor in the city from which you get your bottled water. This company also sent me a list of the added minerals and percentages of each found in the water they bottle and sell. I was told that the water to which the minerals were added was first distilled to remove contaminants and off-flavors. The added minerals present, as stated by an analysis which I have before me, and tested by an independent laboratory include: calcium, magnesium, sodium, potassium, iron, manganese, copper, bicarbonate, chloride, sulfate, nitrate, fluoride (a trace), boron, silica, phosphate. I am purposely not listing the amounts here since the percentages may vary in other bottled waters in other parts of the country. I believe that any consumer can ask the bottling company for the minerals added to water which he is buying and receive the information.

I asked the chemist to whom I spoke if there were other methods of purification besides distillation. He promptly answered: "There are three methods—distillation, reversed osmosis, and de-ionization. I consider de-ionization preferable though we do not use it in all of our plants."

I next asked him if there were any natural springs in the United States still supplying water commercially.

He said yes, that in addition to one well-known one in Arkansas, there were many others throughout the country, most of them small one-to-two-man operations.

Finally I asked him the question: Are we better off with distilled or purified water with added minerals, than natural spring water? He said, "I would not drink natural spring water any longer. If you could see an analysis of such water today it would frighten you because of the pollution." It is his opinion that every stream, every spring large enough to supply many people, and perhaps even a few, is now polluted. Therefore he feels that the treated water is far safer. Then, to my surprise, he added, "If one is drinking straight distilled water that person *must* get added minerals from his diet or supplements or the distilled water will leach the minerals from his own body."

That is exactly what Dr. Nittler and I have been reporting to readers, but coming from the head chemist of a water bottling company, it was a surprise.

On the basis of this information, one must make his own decision on what water to drink. The public health department will usually provide an analysis, when asked, of city water which you drink. If the taste is not offensive (other than chlorine which can be boiled off, or left in the open air to evaporate before refrigerating), then perhaps it is well enough alone. But if the water is fluoridated, or bad-tasting, and otherwise contaminated, distilling plus minerals may be the only solution.

Q. I have an idea, which I hope will be useful. After reading in your column that distilled water leaches the minerals from the body, and not knowing exactly how to compensate for this loss in the body, I wonder if it would not be possible to add to the water the individual cell or tissue salts, in which one may be deficient. Each one of these is an easily assimilated mineral in a sweet-tasting little tablet. What about it?—A.J.G., Columbus, Ohio

A. This question really aroused my interest and I immediately contacted an expert on cell salts to ask his opinion. For those who are newcomers, let me bring you up to date, because the answer to this question is predicated on what has gone before. There has been some information circularized stating that one should not drink hard water because of its effect on hearts, due to the fact that it contains inorganic minerals. This information also states that one should drink distilled water only. I have challenged these statements, due not to the opinion of one person, but to scientists the world over, who believe just the opposite and have proved it with laboratory tests on people and animals. One swallow does not make a summer, nor does one report become a fact.

As I have pointed out many times before, the body needs both inorganic minerals as well as organic minerals and, as proof, on death, the inorganic minerals are always found in the ashes. Furthermore, scientists report that wherever there is *hard water* (which contains inorganic minerals), there is less heart disease. Where there is soft water (with few minerals) or softened water (from a water softener), there is more heart disease. If minerals are not absorbed in the body, but deposited instead in various parts of the body, it is not the fault of the water, but the person who is not assimilating them properly. This is no doubt due, at least in part, to a lack of hydrochloric acid, without which calcium and iron (as well as protein, of course) cannot be dissolved, but piles up in unwanted places.

The Schuessler Cell Salts contain all of the inorganic minerals found in the body. They are easily assimilated without the usual digestion process; they dissolve on the tongue and are absorbed by osmosis. They come separately, or in combination tablets which include them all. I wrote to the expert on these cell salts, thinking that possibly the product which does include them all would be a possible solution to add minerals to distilled water. After all, many people wish to use distilled water to bypass fluoridation, detergents, chlorine and other contamination. The answer I received really shook me up, and should shake you up, too. I will quote from the letter of the expert who lives in one of the largest cities in this country. Now hear this:

"On spending an entire day at our county medical

association library and questioning doctors at our local health department on the subject of distilled water leaching the minerals from the body, one of the doctors verified your remarks on leaching and even stated that a person could actually die as a result of staying on distilled water for an extended period of time.

"An article stated that water with too few minerals [soft water] eats up the plumbing, so imagine what it would do to human plumbing. Also, an article showed that rats given tap water for four weeks showed the least damage, whereas those given distilled water were the most damaged. All but two died.

"As for the complete cell salt product added to a bottle of distilled water, this would be a source of all the minerals, but not practical since there would not be any way of determining just how much water a person would drink each day. Furthermore, the cell salts would not remain in even suspension and a constant shaking would be required, and would give the water a white, murky appearance.

"However, it is particularly important for the person drinking distilled water to take the proper amounts of these cell salts in combination daily to make up for the minerals which have been removed from the water by distillation. These can be taken either according to directions on the bottle, or simply by taking a teaspoonful in the morning."

So those hundreds of people who have written asking how to get their minerals along with their distilled water now know the answer. And so do I, thanks to the person who wrote this question and the expert who answered it.

# WEIGHT

Q. Every time I look around I see another book on losing weight. Magazines are full of articles on losing weight. But nowhere have I found help with my problem, which is a need to gain weight. I am a man and I would like to gain at least 15 pounds. I have been to doctors who have given me all kinds of diets, exercises and drinks to provide more calories, but none have worked. Many people say to eat more of the right foods with more calories and anyone will gain. (Anyone but me, that is.) Doesn't anyone care about underweight people? If I see another book on losing weight I will scream.—J.W., Kansas City, Missouri

A. Dr. Nittler has so wisely said that there are three steps in eating (or taking nutrients): (1) putting them in the mouth (2) digesting them and (3) using them or assimilating them. It appears that your trouble may lie in steps 2 and 3 so let's get to work on that. Do you take extra digestants, particularly hydrochloric acid? Other digestive enzymes including pancreatin and bile salts are worth your consideration, too. Such digestive enzymes are available at health stores.

How is your intestinal flora? One man I know was neither digesting nor assimilating his food properly and had been underweight for over 20 years. He started improving his intestinal flora, particularly with the right type of yogurt (as suggested in an article by Gordon Fraser) as well as taking digestants, such as those already mentioned, and he began to gain weight immediately. He now looks and feels wonderful.

In my opinion, this business of eating more calories to put on more weight, at least for the underweight, is for the birds. High calorie foods are usually the sweets and carbohydrates and not only upset the digestion but put on flabby fat. Protein, on the other hand, enhanced with raw fruits and vegetables (in salads, alone, or in juices) puts on solid, hard, healthy muscles.

Underweight people are usually nervous and tense. This, too, cuts down on proper digestion and assimilation. Do you take enough calcium plus other minerals and B vitamins to keep calm? Please try this complete approach for a while and report the results. We can hardly wait to hear what happens.

Q. I have read all sorts of dire warnings that a high protein, low carbohydrate diet for losing weight can be dangerous. Is this really true?—M.A.W., Greenwich, Connecticut

A. In a study at the Department of Nutrition, Queen Elizabeth College, University of London, Dr. John Yudkin and an associate conducted a study of three men and eight women, aged 21 to 51 years of age. They were given ten to 20 oz. of milk, and as much meat, fish, eggs, cheese, butter, margarine, cream and leafy vegetables daily as they wished. Their daily intake of carbohydrates was limited to 50 grams.

The result of the study is summarized in this statement by the research team: "We conclude that the low carbohydrate diet presents no health hazard, either generally or in regard to its nutritional value. The nutrient content is appreciably higher than could be achieved by a diet in which the same caloric reduction was effected by a general restriction in all foods." (*The American Journal of Clinical Nutrition*, July, 1970.)

Q. Do you gain weight on vitamin and mineral supplements? I get 25,000 units of vitamin A, plus some in my regular diet, daily. I read that an excess of vitamin A is stored in the body.—L.L., Hopkins, Minnesota

A. If there is any excess vitamin A left after your body uses it for its many needs, it is stored (and used as needed) but it is not stored as fat. It is stored in the liver, lungs, skin and eyes and many other areas where it is constantly called upon for maintenance and regeneration of health. Most nutritionists and nutritional physicians do not consider 25,000 units too high for the average person. As far as weight gain is concerned, instead of vitamin and mineral supplements causing weight gain, just the opposite is true. If you were to *eat* the number of calories from food needed to supply the same amount of vitamin/mineral potencies found in supplements, you would have to eat a lot of calories! If you take natural supplements (derived and condensed from natural foods) you can eat less food. Some of all good foods are necessary, but it would take 10 oranges, for example, to supply the amount of vitamin C found in only two 500 mg. tablets. The same amount of vitamins and minerals placed on a small saucer would equal buckets of food.

Q. I have stopped smoking (twice) and each time I gained weight. Isn't getting fat just as bad as tobacco poisoning?—D.F., San Francisco, California

A. Not quite. Smoking has been proved to be a factor in lung cancer. The basic problem is to ask yourself, why do you smoke? Nerves and tension undoubtedly are involved. Calcium, B vitamins and the cell salts nerve combinations (at homeopathic pharmacies and some health stores) can help out here. Sometimes smoking indicates a lack of security; one does not feel at ease under certain situations and smokes to cover it up. Psychologists recognize that in such a case, a smoker reverts to baby habits by sucking something to make him feel comfortable. A cigar as well as a cigarette can fall into this category. Some people smoke because their blood sugar gets low and they feel the need of a pick-up. Eating protein in some form—nuts, cheese, sunflower seeds—instead, will tide you over. Or a tablespoon of brewer's yeast or protein powder stirred into juice or water helps, and the effect lasts a long time.

Once you stop smoking (the hardest part) don't give up too soon. A mere shift from candy to carrot or celery sticks may help, and keep a bit of protein handy in the refrigerator. But here is good news: After-smoking weight gain is fairly common because usually when a person stops smoking, his metabolism slows down. He gains weight even though he may not increase his food intake. However, this is usually temporary, because fortunately, once a person kicks the habit he begins to feel better all over, has more energy and less shortness of breath.

# BEAUTY TIPS

## Hair

Q. Help! Help! I want to be beautiful, too, but between my office job and my home responsibilities, I don't have time. I can't even get to a hairdresser. Isn't there a simple routine I can follow?—A.T., New York City

A. The simplest natural beauty routine I have read for a long time was described in *Vogue,* in June, 1970. An actress told how she cares for her super-sheen, never-set, beautiful chestnut hair. She rubs in warmed olive oil and distributes it through her hair and on her scalp with a plastic scalp massager before shampooing twice weekly. She uses two soapings to remove the oil.

On her face she applies a formula from her grandmother: mix with a fork a raw egg, lemon juice and olive oil and spread on the face to remain for 10 minutes to help tighten pores.

She does her exercises in the bathtub where the warm water helps relax her muscles.

For her nutritional program she steams, not boils, her cooked vegetables, and juices her raw vegetables. For breakfast she puts in a blender orange juice, wheat germ, raw eggs and honey. This, she says, provides her energy.

When asked what makes a woman beautiful, she answered promptly, "Joy, feeling good, active and satisfied."

Such a program takes a minimum of time and should bring a maximum amount of beauty.

Q. My hair is so thin! How can I make it thicker, as it used to be?—B.P., Toledo, Ohio

A. I recently received a letter from a man who has done some further experimenting. He says: "My hair is growing back again. The male pattern baldness (shaped like a receding "M" above the forehead) is slowly going away. I have increased my protein intake, vitamin and mineral intake, use more carrot juice, etc. My supplements are mostly from natural sources. I work on my hair for one hour each day while watching TV—massaging not only the head, but the area from the neck up. My scalp is now loose, hair is growing fast, coming in on the sides and down the center. I have a long way to go but I see definite results. I brush and massage, brush and massage, to step up circulation to the scalp. I even discovered the rolling pin and use that for variety! I'm also using applications of vitamin E since a Japanese experiment states that it makes hair grow 2.4 times faster. This improvement of mine has taken 10 months but it is worth it, and still continuing."

Q. How much vitamin B-2 is safe to take? My 19-year-old granddaughter has unreasonably oily hair. One book says that 5 to 15 mg. will work for this problem, but it has not. She takes 20 mg. of B-2 daily, but has to wash her hair every day since she can almost squeeze the oil out of it. She eats a good diet.—J.C., Lamont, California

A. I cannot prescribe so I cannot say, nor do I know, how much vitamin B-2 your granddaughter needs, or if that is the entire problem. Each person differs. It is true that during the teens oil glands are overactive. Too frequent shampooing, and very hot water overstimulate these glands into secreting even more oil. If shampooing in medium warm water is extended to two days, then three days, and finally to a week apart, the oil glands usually slow down in their manufacture.

I called Jheri Redding on this question. His years in the natural beauty field are unsurpassed, and I (and thousands of beauty salons nationwide) have the greatest respect for his natural beauty knowledge. He advised, for this problem, using an acid-based shampoo (can be ordered by health stores) followed by an Epsom salt rinse. Dissolve 2 tablespoons of Epsom salts to 1 quart of warm water, he said. Towel dry the hair after shampoo and apply this rinse to the hair, but do not wash it off. Set the hair; allow it to dry. Use the rinse every third day, gradually extending it to once a week until the condition improves.

Q. Can dandruff or flaky scalp be caused by nervousness? I take vitamin and mineral supplements daily, use only organic shampoo and use little hair spray, but I do tend to be a nervous person. Also, I would like to know if a person can be allergic to the sun? Every time I am exposed to the sun for even a short time, I break out into itchy bumps. If this is an allergy, what can be done to overcome it? I would like to be at least tanned enough to look healthy.—S.L.S., Portland, Oregon

A. I checked with two physicians. Some people are definitely allergic to sun. Since you mention that you are a nervous person, the physicians (they are both nutritional) wondered if you were getting enough foods and natural supplements which provide B vitamins? I suggest you read and learn everything possible about the entire B complex. The richest food sources are liver, brewer's yeast and wheat germ. Supplements should also include the *entire* B complex, and be derived from natural sources.

The skin and hair can certainly reflect a nervous condition. If your skin responds, why not your scalp, which is part of the skin system? Animals, as well as people, are helped, also, with this dry, flaky condition by taking more unsaturated oils in their diet. For good balance in nutrition, be sure that you have ALL the nutritional substances, not merely a few. Sometimes too much of one B vitamin, for example, may cause a deficiency of another. You need the works!

Sun-worshipping, because it can cause an aging skin as well as skin cancer in some individuals, is going out of style. If you read up and take all the known nutrients, and eat nutritious foods, you should look healthy without being tanned. You will also look younger longer.

Q. Is there any danger in wearing a wig? My hair looks so bad that it is the only solution I have found.—T.O., Hollywood, California

A. One of the best answers to your question I have found comes from Lessie Caraway, who is the owner of a beauty salon near Monterey, California. She says:

"A great danger signal is sweeping America today. I feel we are standing unwisely by and watching the women of this country lose all of their beauty by not explaining to them what can happen to their hair when they do not take proper care of it.

"I feel it will be a sad day when we see ⅔ of the American women having to wear wigs the rest of their lives. A woman should wear a wig, at the most, 3 days a week, but I find women wearing wigs from 48 to 65 hours per week. This cannot go on for too long a time without some permanent damage and that's when the sad time will be. It makes no difference how strong grass on a lawn might be. If you turn a pail down over it and let it stay one month, it will kill the roots of the grass.

"Well, the hair on the head is a little stronger than that, but don't tell yourself you can wear a wig 10 and 12 hours a day. I feel it just won't work. I feel that if a woman starts wearing a wig every day, 8 to 12 hours per day, by the time she does this 8 to 10 years, the actual texture of her hair will change and diminish. I feel if a woman begins wearing a wig steadily at the age of 23, by the time she is 35, her hair may have the appearance of an 80-year-old woman.

"One of the things to keep in mind is that people who have studied and worked with wigs do not have a collection of wigs themselves. As they learn about wigs, they become acquainted with all the phases, good and bad, of wearing wigs too often."

Q. Is there any substitute for false eyelashes? They are so much trouble to apply.—G.C., Denver, Colorado

A. Yes. Emily Wilkins, in her book, *A New You* (a book for teen-agers, published by Putnam and Co.), suggests a method which can work for adults, too. She writes, "False eyelashes may cause your own eyelashes to fall out. Every time you glue them on and pull them off you are courting trouble. Instead, you can produce the look of false eyelashes with this method: Coat your lashes with mascara. Apply a little powder to the tips of the lashes with a cotton swab. Recoat with mascara. Repeat, if necessary. The result: fantastic, fluttery eyelashes."

## Face

Q. I am a dietitian. I would like to know what can be done for the prevention of whiteheads on the face. I have consulted specialists but none were able to answer. I am very anxious to know.—Mrs. F.U., Fort Lee, New Jersey

A. I went to my oracle of natural beauty, Jheri Redding, for help with this problem. This is what he said: A whitehead is sebaceous material which is caught by or in a membrane in the subcutaneous layer of the skin. Since it cannot come all the way through, it becomes a whitehead. To eliminate it, soften and deep cleanse the skin in order that this bit of sebaceous material can get all the way through—and off! To do this, Mr. Redding advises to keep the skin softened with any unsaturated vegetable oil, day and night for four or five days. This will soften the under cuticle and allow the whitehead to finally push through and be eliminated. From then on, he added, keep your skin well cleansed to allow body oil and dirt to come through the pores easily. Taking vitamin C and E also has an effect on keeping the skin in a healthy condition in this problem.

Q. Is deep massage good for the face and neck?—B.L., Wichita, Kansas

A. A new book, *How to Use Your Hands to Help Your Face*, by Jessica Krane (Information Inc., New York, N.Y., 1969), states that heavy-handed massage can play havoc with your face. Miss Krane says rough or heavy massage will eventually break down the skin, tissues and musculature to the point that they can never be restored to normal. As a former concert pianist and a teacher of hundreds of classes of men and women in her method, called "Face-o-Metrics," she advises a pianissimo (very soft) touch in smoothing cosmetics onto the skin. She feels that only gentle stroking relaxes the face so that lines seem to disappear of their own accord. She warns against touching the skin under your eyes with any pressure at all. "Leave it alone" she warns. Finger contact in cleansing or applying under eye make-up should be no heavier than a mere whisper, an art which must be learned.

Q. Is there a face exercise to plump out the cheeks and mouth of a person whose teeth have been pulled?—K.B., Granger, Washington

A. Any exercise which will bring fresh circulation to the face will help. Make a tight oval of the mouth and then try to stretch (while holding the oval) all the muscles of the face in a sunburst pattern outward and *away* from the oval. Several times night and morning will help the mouth and cheeks feel warm, showing that the circulation to those areas has been encouraged.

Nutrients help, too, as you will see in my book, *Secrets of Health and Beauty.* Protein vegetable oils and lecithin added to the diet help to keep the tissues under the surface of the cheek and mouth area firm.

Q. I am going to be 69 soon. I have a pretty good skin for my age, but the thing that worries me most are the lines around my mouth. They make me very self-conscious. Is there anything I can do to make them disappear or appear less conspicuous? I do wear dentures, but so does my husband. Though he is older he doesn't have these wrinkles.—Mrs. O.C., Cleveland, Ohio

A. The lines around your mouth are no doubt due to poor muscle tone in that area, causing the tissues to shrink and wrinkle. This would indicate that these muscles need more protein. To plump them up from the inside, increase your protein intake via your diet, being sure that you have enough hydrochloric acid to help digest and utilize it. (This may well be the difference between you and your husband. Even though you eat the same diet, he may be assimilating his protein better than you).

Vitamin B-2 often helps this condition, too.

To plump up the tissues from the outside, apply the liquid collagenous protein for cosmetic purposes. To 3 oz. of any type of unsaturated vegetable oil, add 1 oz. of the protein. Stir before each use. Rub in and leave all night. Health stores can at last definitely get this collagenous protein.

Finally, use an exercise daily to help strengthen the muscles and tighten them so that the wrinkles will be helped to smooth out. Make an O with your mouth and tense *hard* several times until you feel all the area around your mouth tighten and fresh circulation warming it up.

## HELP FOR SCOWL LINES

Q. Can you give me an exercise to reduce or eliminate a scowl line?—A.B., Columbus, Ohio

A. Marjorie Craig's book has an exercise for the scowl line. To lessen lines between the eyebrows, she says, "Start with eyes wide open, then pull brows down over the eyes in a real frown. Frown even harder; then lift the eyebrows as high as you can, at the same time opening your eyes as wide as you can. Frown-and-lift 5 times."

Another exercise is: Sit at a table or desk. Put your right elbow on the surface of the table or desk and then rest the frown area against the heel of your right hand. Now push the frown lines against the heel of your hand. Don't let the *hand* do the pushing; let the frown area push against your hand! This strengthens these face muscles themselves. After you have done this several times, then use compression. Here's how: Use the soft pads of your three middle finger tips. Press the frown area and let go. Press and let go. Do this several times. This compression method really brings the blood to the surface you wish to smooth and helps to plump up the skin at that point. Physiotherapists often use this method to bring fresh blood to a lazy or sluggish part of the body. But don't delude yourself that these exercises will cure unless you use prevention, too. Frowning is a habit and each time you frown it deepens the crease in your skin.

To help remember not to frown, as well as smooth away a frown line for a while, use Arlene Dahl's suggestion of putting Scotch magic tape on your frown area while you work or while you sleep. It's a real help.

Q. After an operation some years ago, my doctor prescribed some hormones which caused thick hair growth on my upper lip. This hair growth was removed by electrolysis, but probably weakened the muscles. Consequently, deep vertical lines developed. Can anything be done to eliminate them?—Miss A., New Orleans, Louisiana

A. There are two avenues to follow here: One, increase the use of protein in your diet to help rebuild both skin and muscles (skin is about 95 percent protein). The other is to use a mouth exercise to strengthen the muscles in that area. Make an "O" with your lips. Holding your cheeks and upper lip areas taut, make this "O" bigger and wider as if you were saying "Wow," against the strong resistance of the entire lower part of your face. You will feel the circulation increasing in these areas, and thus the blood stream can help nourish and strengthen the area you wish to improve.

Q. I have been on a nutritional program for years. It has included vitamins, minerals, fruits and raw vegetables. As I get older, my upper lip is getting wrinkles. Why?

Also, what is a good exercise to reduce hips?—M.E.J., Atlanta, Georgia

A. You do not mention protein in your nutritional program. Not only is skin nearly 98% protein, but the muscles which support it are also made of protein. When protein is undersupplied to the body, the results are not noticeable at first, but flabbiness and wrinkles become apparent as one ages and the deficiency increases. Adding protein to the diet to help regenerate the muscles under your lip, and in other facial areas, and applying protein in some form to the skin itself, will help. Collagenous protein liquid for skin and hair application is becoming available in health stores. Read and follow the directions.

One more thing: Place the fingertips of both hands on your upper lip to hold it firm, then try to make a wide "O," pulling inwards and outwards with your mouth against the resistance of your fingertips. Repeat several times to bring circulation to the lip area.

Debbie Drake suggests this exercise for hip reducing: Stand with your hands on your hips. Cross the right leg over the left knee and as you step forward, bend your knee as far as you can. Now cross the left leg over the right knee with another deep knee bend. Do this exercise as a walk, starting with a few steps and increasing the number each day. According to Debbie Drake, you will feel the pull as this firms, slims, shapes and trims the hips. She also suggests walking, stair-climbing, and bicycling for improving hips and thighs. Golf and tennis are means of having fun and improving your figure at the same time.

## Skin

Q. What causes large pores? What can I do to make them smaller?—Mrs. M.E.L., Cincinnati, Ohio

A. Large pores indicate a lack of tensile strength in the muscles around the pore itself. Two methods may be used to correct this condition: helping to rebuild the muscle by applying protein (of which muscle is made) and using a tightening substance as well. A liquid protein is available in some beauty salons and is also becoming available in health stores. This substance can be applied to the skin as a night treatment, according to the directions which accompany it. Witch hazel can be smoothed on during the daytime as a tightener. For faster results, rubbing your face with an ice cube or so, wrapped in a cloth, may help.

Above all, cleanse your face every eight hours! The

debris that is constantly expelled through the skin (though invisible to you) should not be allowed to remain in the pores to stretch them.

Q. I have oily skin and tend to get enlarged pores, although I wash frequently and use an astringent. Is there anything else I can do to minimize this problem? Also, would you recommend the use of mayonnaise on the face (or hair) as described in your book, *Secrets of Health and Beauty,* when the condition is so oily to begin with?—W.H., Long Beach, California

A. I asked Jheri Redding, because of his many years of experience in the natural beauty field, for help with this question. Here is his answer: "Mix three parts of collagenous protein with one part of distilled water and apply as you would a cream. (This mixture should be refrigerated and will last for three weeks.)

"Research points to the fact that the addition of the B vitamins, particularly B-6, pantothenic acid as well as vitamin A taken daily, are extremely beneficial. It would be advisable to keep on using the mayonnaise as it is also beneficial for this condition."

Q. I am allergic to commercial deodorants and break out in a rash when I use them. Are there any available which do not contain the aluminum sulfate which I think is what causes my problem?—M.H., Kansas City, Missouri

A. You can find a deodorant at health stores which is free from this or other chemical additives, or watch the mail order ads for one which is so gentle that no one I know who has used it has had any unpleasant reaction. It contains no irritants at all. Chemically the active ingredients are from the borated soda family—making the deodorant cream effective and harmless. It can even be used on the hands to deodorize them after cutting onions!

Q. For a number of years I have been bothered with very dry skin on my lower lip only, with little flakes of the dry skin constantly forming, which makes the lip very rough. I have applied castor oil, wheat germ oil and many of the vegetable and seed oils from the health food stores with no results. Is there anything I can do to correct this condition?—J.K.R., Hollywood, California

A. I called on two experts in this field. One was Katie Pugh, author of *Hair Thru Diet,* as well as Jheri Redding, who knows so much about skin problems. I asked Katie because she mentions in her book that after using a photo-sensitive lipstick, her own lips peeled for two or three years. She said: "To heal the scalds and burns of the lipstick, I worked from the inside mostly. I took large amounts of B complex, plus extra B-2, plus other B complex any way I could get it, including liquid form. I also took natural oils. I used no lipstick for over three years. Just applying something on the lips never worked. I tried for months that way. It was only after the above routine that they healed. To keep the lips from cracking I used a natural lip pomade stick."

Jheri concurred with this approach. He also advocated vitamin B for the condition. And while I had him on the phone I asked what to do for hangnails. He advised vitamin E.

Q. I have ugly stretch marks on my breasts, hips and thighs as a result of an extensive weight loss. I acquired them three years ago. Is there anything I can take internally or apply externally to erase these marks?—L.S., Long Beach, California

A. Our grandmothers used cocoa butter (available in drug and some health stores). They rubbed it on their stretch marks which followed childbirth and the marks disappeared. Remember, too, that skin is about 97 per cent protein. If you are deficient in protein or in hydrochloric acid (which helps your body assimilate protein), adding both to your diet should help. Many people state that taking a heaping tablespoon of protein powder in juice once or twice daily, in addition to using protein at every meal, has helped them to become firm.

An anthropologist from the University of California, Dr. R. D. McCracken, recently told the American Anthropological Association that "man is basically a meat- and fruit-eating animal. The carbohydrate or starches are an unnatural diet for him. Carbohydrates make sugar more easily absorbed by the body and upset delicate body chemistries. Proteins are eventually converted to sugar but much more slowly and safely." Carbohydrates also tend to make one flabby, which can lead to loose skin.

Q. In the past five years many brown spots have appeared on the backs of my hands, and now are appearing on my face, high up on my cheeks. I have consulted several specialists but none have been able to give the cause or the remedy. I should appreciate any suggestions.—Mrs. J.N.M., Odessa, Texas

A. Quoting one expert, "You cannot have a clear skin if your intestines are clogged with poisons and toxins, which lead to a toxic liver. . . . Brown spots on hands or face are merely a sign that poisons have piled up in the intestines and liver." The woman who made this statement has a beautiful, clear, pink-and-white skin.

Adelle Davis has said that taking vitamin E helps to fade spots in some (not all) people. Others advocate applying vitamin E or castor oil directly to the spots. I recently investigated an English product (not available yet in this country) which helped many people who rubbed it on the spots. The product contains sulfur.

## Eyes and Nails

Q. What can I do to lengthen and strengthen my fingernails?— V.W., Los Angeles, California

A. I have mentioned bone meal before. According to Alfred Aslander, Ph.D., of Sweden, this should be *true* bone meal, not bone ash, which he believes is not fit for human consumption. He says you can tell the difference easily: bone ash is chalk white, looks like chalk, but with no taste or odor. True bone meal, he says, is somewhat yellow in color and has a faint animal taste and odor. It contains more nutrients and minerals in addition to the calcium. People who take it regularly report stronger teeth, bones and fingernails.

Another help: a reader recently wrote me that she experienced the first real growth of fingernails in her lifetime as a result of eating a few fresh comfrey leaves daily. The leaves—if young—can be added to salads or if they are larger can be blended in a blender into a juice or health drink together with other ingredients of your choice.

Q. What causes fingernail ridges? I am 52 years old, teach school, and am under pressure and strain a lot. The ridges started several years ago.—O.G., Dallas, Texas

A. You did not say whether the ridges were horizontal or longitudinal. Horizontal ridges are formed during menstruation. Longitudinal ridges are a result of anemia. Be sure you include in your diet, liver (fresh or desiccated) and other natural sources of iron (ask your health store) as well as generous portions of protein, of which nails are largely made.

Q. I will soon be 50 and my eyelids are getting so baggy. What causes this? Can anything be done to keep them from getting worse? Do face exercises help?—Mrs. E., Miami, Florida

A. Marjorie Craig, in her book, *Miss Craig's Face Saving Exercises* (Random House, N.Y.C., November, 1970), gives a corrective exercise for this condition, which is no doubt due to weak muscles and perhaps too little protein. She advises: "Looking into a mirror, tightly place thumb and index finger on inside corners of eyes. Close your eyes. Then squeeze the corners of your eyes in *toward your fingers* (first position). When you think you have squeezed as hard as you can, squeeze even harder (second position). S-l-o-w-l-y release the squeeze. Do the entire exercise three times.

Q. What causes dark circles under the eyes? How can I get rid of them?—E.H.J., Washington, D.C.

A. Dark circles can be caused by an allergy. This is often the case in people who are using a commercial hair dye or tint. Actually, since a chemical in the hair dye (or even a cosmetic) may be the cause, the body, particularly the liver, needs help in detoxifying.

But there is another surprising cause of dark circles. I have never seen a person with a parasite (intestinal) infestation who did not have dark circles. In fact, in members of my own family who lived in India, where intestinal parasites are common, I have found a perfect correlation between dark circles and parasites. When the parasites were routed, the circles disappeared. Your doctor can make a test to see if you have them and give you the proper remedy.

Q. What can I do for very swollen, puffy eyelids on arising every morning? The swelling lasts for several hours, sometimes most of the day. I am in my late 40's and my doctor tells me I am in very good health.—Mrs. J.H., San Jose, California

A. Eye puffiness can come from excessive water retention, which, if your doctor has ruled out kidney disturbance, might yield to a natural diuretic, such as vitamin B-6, vitamin C, or magnesium; or it can be caused by a deficiency of protein.

Most likely, though, you are suffering from an allergy. What do you put on your face the night before? Eliminate it and see if it does not disappear. It might even be an allergy to pillows, bedding or some environmental situation. Do a little detective work until you find, and eliminate, the culprit.

# THE HOUSEHOLD



Q. What types of kitchen utensils are unsafe?—M.J., Fayetteville, North Carolina

A. Since so many people ask me this question, I will tell you what I use. I use glass, as well as the milky glassware which is impervious to high heat or freezing cold and breaks only if you drop it. I also love cast-iron and enameled iron—unless the enamel begins to chip, in which case I discard it. I do not use aluminum as a result of the incriminating evidence I have read. For other types of utensils I am going to include here the excellent answers from Margaret Dana, a food expert, which appeared in the *San Francisco Chronicle* several years ago.

"There are cast-iron skillets that have well served several generations of cooks. They were never dropped (cracks would probably result), and the built-up "seasoning" of cooking surfaces through slow absorption of fats and oils was never disturbed by scouring. So rust never attacked the iron.

"Stainless steel is given high marks for durability, but to earn these it must be good-quality stainless steel. According to the Committee of Stainless Steel Producers of the American Iron and Steel Institute, stainless steel properly is a solid alloy that must contain at least 11½ per cent of chromium in order to qualify as "stainless." Unfortunately, since the import door was recently opened wider—to permit more stainless steel products to enter at lower tariffs—there is an increasing amount of so-called stainless steel, especially from Japan, which may or may not meet this standard.

"The older, gray enameled ware contained an antimony compound in its manufacture. This is poisonous when in contact with food. The director of the Bureau of Food Control of Baltimore assures me this is no longer generally available, but some pieces may still be around our kitchens. You may have inherited some, or your church kitchen may have had some stored for years. It should be discarded.

"The second hazard comes from utensils apparently made during World War II when aluminum was scarce and substitutes were used. Cadmium was one of those substitutes, since it has a silvery color like aluminum. It is no longer being sold, according to the Baltimore Health Department, but some may still be in kitchens here and there.

"I was told how, during World War II, an entire battleship was put out of action—not by the enemy, but by a quantity of fruit gelatine (an acid food) prepared in cadmium trays and served aboard ship. Apparently the food poisoning from the cadmium does not always occur (doubtless only with acid foods) or we should have heard about it more often.

"The third hazard arises from the misuse of a container not intended for food. Suppose, for instance, a committee or a hostess was preparing food for a crowd and had no container big enough in which to make fruit punch. A nice new, or scoured, galvanized garbage can might seem just the thing. Don't use it. It becomes dangerous if used for the preparation of acid-type foods like lemonade or punch. Any food acid actually etches the zinc from the surface of the container and deposits it in the food or drink. Known cases of such zinc poisoning are on record.

"Finally, there is a warning that unglazed ceramics as containers for acid-type foods can also create dangers. It appears that lead, a component of the pottery material, is absorbed by foods stored in unglazed ceramics. When glazed, as most pottery and china is, food is protected from the lead. But it was found, for instance, that cole-slaw left in unglazed pottery jars a few hours will absorb enough lead to be poisonous."

Q. Is Teflon safe to use?—Mrs. H.E.K., Battle Lake, Minnesota

A. Teflon can be extremely dangerous unless certain precautions are observed, which many people can't or won't bother to take. As proof, several years ago a large aircraft, missile and spacecraft company (whose name I am purposely not mentioning to protect them from pressure from industrial vested interests) sent out a warning against Teflon, complete with documentation. The report points out that because it is extremely resistant to corrosive chemicals, Teflon was originally used in industry for wire insulation, limiter blocks, electrical applications, chemical containers and equipment, before it invaded the household. As long as Teflon remains unheated, no human disturbances have been noted. But the minute it gets hot, watch out!

The report states: "Toxic gases from heated Teflon can cause serious illness when significant amounts are inhaled into the respiratory system. The illness generally takes a form similar to influenza, causing chills, shakes, fever, and headache. In such cases, medical care is necessary."

When Teflon is heated above 500 degrees, toxic gases are produced. In the factory this can occur during soldering, molding, heating, high speed machining and grinding. Such danger can also come from Teflon-coated ovens and furnaces which may reach 500 degrees or more. In the home, when a Teflon-coated pan is left forgotten on a hot burner, or an iron sits unattended on a Teflon-coated ironing board cover, there is potential danger for the entire family.

The report warns, "In the factory, cigarettes or other tobacco products carried in the pocket in the work area should be covered in order to prevent contamination with Teflon dust or particles. Avoid burning Teflon scraps in incinerators and furnaces unless the fumes are vented and mechanical draft is provided. The disposal of Teflon scrap should be preferably buried in the ground or at a dump.

"DO NOT BREATHE THE FUMES ARISING FROM HEATING OF TEFLON IN ANY CIRCUMSTANCES," the report concludes.

In one medical journal, the story is told of a factory worker who left a burning cigarette on a sheet of Teflon. He had to be rushed to a hospital to save his life from breathing the fumes. A housewife who leaves a lighted cigarette on a Teflon-coated ironing board cover runs the same risk as the factory worker.

Teflon is the trade name for fluorocarbon resins. It is used as a coating and produces a wax-like finish. Although there are not yet any reports of illness resulting from the chips or grains which are loosened from a pan after stirring, those loosened particles, evident by the scarred surface which eventually develops on the inside surface of the pan, have to go *somewhere,* most likely into the food and then into the stomach. There are too many potential hazards of Teflon to recommend its use.

Documentation:
1. "Teflon Fluorocarbon Resins and Their Decomposition Products," American Industrial Hygiene Association, 14125 Prevost, Detroit, Mich. 48227. *Hygiene Guide,* April 1963.
2. "Industrial Hazards Control Bulletin No. 3," The Boeing Co., Industrial Relations Department, Seattle, Wash. (April 1961).
3. "Handling and Use of Teflon Fluorocarbon Resins at High Temperatures," E. I. duPont De Nemours & Co., Polychemicals Dept., Wilmington, Delaware 19898.

Q. I have some attractive Mexican pottery I bought recently on a vacation in Mexico. It gives off a peculiar odor. I am wondering if it is safe to put food in it.—Mrs. I.B., Tacoma, Washington

A. The FDA has recently warned that Mexican pottery or earthenware should not be used for cooking, storing or serving food, because of the possibility of lead poisoning. The odor—or the lack of it—should not be used as a guide. The FDA said that 26 out of 28 different samples of Mexican cookware were found to contain lead in varying amounts, leached from the glaze. Importers and distributors of Mexican cookware have been informed that their products must be recalled and examined by the FDA.

Q. I am using a product which is sprayed onto a pan for cooking foods so that butter or cooking oils are not needed. The listed ingredients stated on the label are lecithin and propellants. What are propellants? Are they considered as possibly dangerous?—P.D., New Orleans, Louisiana

A. A propellant is a gas in an aerosol container which propels or pushes out the contents at the push of the finger. There are different types of gas used, and the industry is very quiet about them all. The only one to be *proved* dangerous to date was one used in hair sprays and which included PVP, an ingredient which, according to Dr. Wilhelm Hueper (formerly at the National Cancer Institute), can cause malignant growths. In a year-long study at a St. Louis Hospital lymph nodes in lungs of women were traced to the hair spray. When the women stopped using the sprays, the abnormalities gradually cleared up. The California Medical Association has issued these warnings about hair spray, due to the propellant:

* Spray on only the amount necessary to keep the hair under control.
* Direct the spray as far away from the nose and mouth as possible.
* Take deep breaths before releasing hair spray and then limit your breathing.
* Move to another room before taking another deep breath.
* Ascertain, if possible, whether the spray contains plastic material and if so, be doubly cautious.

This does not mean that all gas propellants are necessarily harmful, but one allergist states that the same compressed gas used as a refrigerant, which during a slow leak has caused chronic symptoms for highly susceptible people, could have similar effects when released from an aerosol can or spray container dispensing perfume, hair spray and other products.

Since most people do not get enough fats in their diet, a small amount of butter or vegetable oil, if not allowed to smoke, will neither cause trouble nor add weight for reducers, so why use a gas propellant in the first place? There are hair sprays, perfumes and other products which can be released from a container by air pressure, like an atomizer, which do not need a gas propellant. I vote for this type.

Q. What about using the product for frying that they claim has almost as much left after the food is fried as there was at the start? Is it good to use from the calorie standpoint? Also, what about "instantized flour"—we all know it is a poor substitute for whole grain flours—but it is convenient to use occasionally.—Mrs. R.A.K., San Diego, California

A. The brand of fat you mention is considered one of the hydrogenated fats. Such fats provide calories but no health values. As Adelle Davis says, "Unfortunately food manufacturers have become hydrogenation-happy. Each year the list grows longer and longer. French dressing, mayonnaise and salad oil appear to be the only good sources of the valuable essential fatty acids [unsaturated, unhydrogenated] left."

A hydrogenated fat is a saturated fat, and there has been much speculation that the saturated fats may lead to heart disease. In saturated fats, lecithin (a normal dissolver of cholesterol) and some B vitamins have been removed. Adelle Davis suggests that if you wish to reduce or maintain your weight to eat *at least* two tablespoons of vegetable fat daily. Vegetable fats are unsaturated fats and thus safer. So it is not a question of how much fat is left on the food after frying with any saturated fat, nor even the number of calories, but the bad effect of saturated or hydrogenated fat you do eat! Use vegetable oil for frying.

So that I will not be tempted, I do not allow a hydrogenated fat, white sugar or white flour in my house! I cook with vegetable oil. I sweeten with a little raw sugar or honey. I use unbleached flour. Instantized flour has also been tampered with, removing valuable nutrients, and every bit counts of whatever food you eat. If you want to use a small, convenient thickener, without worrying about flour lumps, as in a white sauce or gravy, try arrowroot. It is a natural product, looks and acts and feels like cornstarch but is safer. You will find it in most food stores on shelves with the seasonings.

Q. Is it true that it is dangerous to mix cleaning agents?—H.T., Omaha, Nebraska

A. It apparently is very dangerous. Breathing any strong cleaning agent can be a hazard in itself. One woman whose head was inside her oven while using an oven cleaner was asphyxiated and had to be taken to the hospital to recover. Other cases have been cited which indicate that by combining two household cleaners, there is even more danger because a poisonous gas is liberated when two cleaning agents are mixed. For instance, there have been reports that housewives who combined an ordinary bathroom bowl cleaner with a common household bleach either died or were hospitalized for several weeks. A U.S. Navy medical newsletter reported the cases of 20 people who were felled with gases resulting from mixing a chlorine bleach and ammonia. Chlorine should not be used with any other cleaning agent including bathroom bowl cleaners, ammonia, lye, rust removers, vinegar or oven cleaner, according to this Navy medical newsletter.

Ann Landers reported this danger, too, and I hope everyone sees it.

Q. What kind of toothpaste is best?

A. Usually the toothpastes you find at health stores. There are many commercial brands which make all sorts of claims, now seriously being questioned. If you have noticed a biting or stinging sensation in a toothpaste it might be due to chloroform, according to a report in *Consumer's Bulletin* of April, 1969. The article also said that the American Dental Association now accepts baking soda as a toothpaste. Some people combine salt and soda. We all know that children, however, depend upon a good flavor in a toothpaste.

Q. It seems to me that I spend most of my life in my kitchen. Although it is really pleasant, with cheerful fluorescent lighting, no housewife wants to be chained to nonstop cooking, dishwashing, etc., etc., no matter how convenient. With my large family I have little choice. What really worries me is that, probably because I don't get outside enough, my skin is becoming more and more blemished. Can you suggest help?—I.K., Cambridge, Massachusetts

A. That word "fluorescent" in your question caught my eye. Although I, too, have fluorescent fixtures in my kitchen, Dr. John Ott woke me up to their hazards. (His article appears in *Let's LIVE,* October, 1969.) I replaced the bulbs with the ones he recommends, as listed at the end of the article—item #2.

Barbara Cartland, writing in the English health magazine, *Here's Health* (Feb., 1970), tells of a client who had skin trouble similar to yours. Miss Cartland learned that the young woman worked in an office with fluorescent lighting. She told her that fluorescents take the vitamin A out of the skin and suggested that she should add vitamin A generously to her diet and in supplement form. A week later the woman returned with a perfectly clear skin! If this seems miraculous, *Vogue* (April 1, 1970) states that skin cells shed and regenerate to produce a new surface every 18 hours. If they are cleansed and properly fed with repair material, healing is hastened.

The skin is not alone in reacting against fluorescents. Two of my friends worked in different fluorescent-lighted banks. They both developed eye trouble, another indication of vitamin A deficiency.

Q. Are sun lamps harmful or beneficial? I am a part-time secretary and have to spend two days a week in an office where there are no windows at all and fluorescent tubes are being used. You have reported that Dr. John Ott, the expert on the effect of different types of light on health, calls fluorescents harmful to health and eyes. I would like to find an office where I would find daylight, but such offices are not easy to find in this city. Meanwhile I am taking multiple vitamins and minerals, extra cod liver oil, vitamin C, B complex, dolomite, bone meal tablets, magnesium oxide and B-6. I also take brewer's yeast, acidophilus, bifidus (for intestinal flora) and I drink carrot juice. Dr. Ott recommends Vita Light fluorescent tubes which are close to daylight and therefore not harmful. We do not have these tubes in my office and the boss does not want to have them installed. Is the use of sun lamps helpful for this lack of daylight and what should I add to my diet in order to be completely protected?—J.J., New York City

A. I am sorry that your boss is disinterested in the safe daylight tubes for fluorescent fixtures in your office. After reading Dr. Ott's research I changed immediately to them in my kitchen and I am delighted with them. I wrote to Dr. Ott, who is head of the Environmental Health and Light Research Institute, for help with your question. He considers it tragic that so many buildings are without windows and have fluorescent lighting which he says is "definitely harmful." The safe tubes are quite inexpensive and every office would be wise to make the change-over. Dr. Ott tells of instances where tempers also became frayed under fluorescent lighting and were restored to normal as soon as the safe tubes were substituted.

Dr. Ott wrote me: "The so-called sun lamps are dangerous when used except under the supervision of professionals." He suggests that you spend as much time outdoors as possible, use good lighting in your home, and—if possible—change jobs.

Your diet sounds excellent. I do not see any vitamin A listed but assume it is contained in the multiple vitamin-mineral supplement. I wish more people were as alert to environmental problems and willing to do something constructive.

Q. I have heard that anything in a spray can is dangerous, whether it's hair spray, room deodorizers (I don't use pesticides), or perfume, even cleaning agents, because of the gas in the can which propels the substance out in the air. Is this true?—M.B., Kansas City, Missouri

A. Indeed it is. Jack Anderson, in his courageous column, *Merry-Go-Round,* states that these sprayers can become a blowtorch if used near a flame, and contain chemicals such as polymers, plasticizers, solvents, as well as scents, *in addition* to the gas or propellant, which can be dangerous for the eyes, the lungs, mucous membranes, and the heart.

The most common propellant is Freon, originally used only for refrigeration. Tests show that hearts of animals have suffered damage from this dangerous product and I do not have to remind you that many children who have inhaled the spray for "kicks" have died. One child in my community is still living after inhaling spray which had been pumped into a paper sack, but he is now mentally retarded and, according to doctors, will remain so the rest of his life. There are safer sprays, without gas propellants, which require a little finger-pumping action—but well worth the effort!

Q. In the February, 1971, *Let's LIVE* (letters section) a reader gave some tips for controlling household pests—boric acid to stop roaches, and pepper for ants. I live in Florida and this is a big problem. We have had an exterminator for the past four years on a monthly basis for regular pests as well as to control fleas and ticks. (We have two dogs and two cats.) I am becoming increasingly concerned about the build-up for all of us, including the pets. We plan to stop the exterminator in the fall, when the bugs are not as bad. Can you give any other harmless suggestions for controlling pests?—P.H., Deerfield Beach, Florida

A. This is a real problem, worse in some states than others. I, too, am concerned about the products exterminators use and refuse to have one for the same reasons you give. Let's start with pets first. There is a one-spot flea-killer powder which is applied on a small area at the back of the neck of the animal for fleas, ticks and lice. It is made of rotenone and considered safe. You can find it at pet stores. My vet sold me a spray for the same purposes, though the ingredients sound somewhat forbidding. It does work, but perhaps needs caution and fewer applications.

For other pests, including roaches and ants, someone has suggested putting a pathway of ordinary sink cleansing powder on the ant or roach runway, or for sweet-eating ants, mixing the powder with honey. You can also buy Driedie or diatomacious earth, often from health stores. These powders stop the breathing of the pests as they walk through them.

A service known as Concern, Inc., 2100 M Street N.W.,

Washington, D.C. 20037, gives the following suggestions. Try pyrethrin-based sprays (made from a type of daisy), safe in themselves, though often combined with dangerous additives in some products. Rotenone is a related and safe product, providing it is not combined with dangerous additives. Concern, Inc., suggests the following pyrethrin-based sprays: Raid House and Garden Bug Killer; Raid Flying Insect Killer; D-Con Ant and Fly Spray; D-Con Warpath; Hot Shot Fly and Mosquito Spray; Hot Shot House and Garden Pest Killer; Johnston's No-Roach Spray.

I have found Amazon insect killer for flies, roaches, moths, mosquitos, ants and worms, excellent. It is made from mineral oil, sesame oil, pyrethrins and inert ingredients. (Tro Chemical Works, Inc., Brooklyn, New York.)

Concern, Inc., warns against no-pest strips, particularly in the kitchen, shelf- or wall-paper treated with pesticides, and I guess everybody knows of deaths caused by lindane bug vapor killers (or any other type of vapor killer). Concern, Inc., adds, "If you feel you must call an exterminator, insist that he use the safest possible sprays." However, the double talk I have often heard from some of these exterminators is that there is no danger in any pesticide.

**Q. Recently I heard that cooking with charcoal is more dangerous than smoking cigarettes. Will you please comment?—J.L.E., Evadale, Texas**

A. There have been many reports of the dangers of charcoal cooking. The reason given is that the hot fat falling from the meat onto the coals is burned and the smoke carries the carbon upward to the meat, coating it. For those who enjoy charcoal cookery (and who doesn't) there is an excellent solution. There are available on the market some upright charcoal cookers. An old-fashioned toaster rack, which holds the meat, hangs from hooks in *front* of (not above) the hot charcoal and the smoke, which rises, does not contaminate the meat, which is to one side. There are other charcoal cookers with a slanted run-off pan by the charcoal so that the melting fat is carried away from the coals before it has a chance to burn. Please do not write and ask me where to get these cookers because I do not know. I have seen them, and used the upright variety myself, and find it highly satisfactory. I got mine years ago from a hardware section of a large department store. Perhaps hardware store catalogues can help you.

# MISCELLANEOUS

## TENSION

Q. I am a working girl. When I drive, or work long hours at my desk, my neck muscles get awfully tense. Is there anything I can do to relieve this tension?—F.H., Brownsville, Texas

A. Stretching the back of your neck often helps. One of the easiest ways to relieve neck tension and congestion is to pull in your chin several times daily. As you draw your chin in, the muscles at the back of your neck are automatically stretched.

This is important for other reasons, too. If you keep your head constantly bent forward, it creates a barrier to the circulation of blood to your neck and head. James and Leslie Thomson, authors of the book, *Healthy Hair,* remind you to straighten up often. They state that upright posture of the neck may improve the circulation of nutrition to the scalp more than any other treatment. It is only logical that this would also apply to eyes, and even to the brain. So pull in your chin and stretch your neck often.

## FIBERGLASS FILLINGS

Q. Do you have any information about the new fiberglass dental fillings?—D.P., Indianapolis, Indiana

A. Yes, I have a friend who just tried them. Although his experience may differ from that of others, this is what happened to him after acquiring three small fillings of this supposedly "better" material. He experienced excess salivation and eye watering; irritation in his trachea requiring constant clearing of throat and light coughing to bring up mucous; depressed heart action; and a feeling of tension. Apparently, according to my friend, who is a professional physical diagnostician, the fiberglass seems to be an irritant to the para-sympathetic nervous system.

At any rate, after a week of this suffering, he went back to the dentist, had the fiberglass fillings removed and replaced with silver. All unpleasant symptoms stopped.

Warnings against contact with fiberglass in fabrics have already been sounded. This is the first I have heard about disturbing reactions in the mouth.

## INCREASING BUSTLINE

Q. Is there any way to increase the bustline? I've heard that vitamin E can help, as well as exercises.—A.A., Anchorage, Alaska

A. Perhaps vitamin E will help, though I have seen no scientific reports. Applications of cocoa butter were used by our grandmothers. One nutritionist has conducted studies in which lecithin redistributed weight throughout the body and, in some cases, improved the bustline. However, exercise has really proved to be a safe and helpful method. One isometric exercise is easy and has been found rewarding by many, whether it is a do-it-yourself technique or done with an exerciser which I described in my book, *Secrets of Health and Beauty*. Before-and-after pictures apparently testify to this success. The exercise: Put the heel of one palm crosswise against the heel of the other. With bent elbows, holding your arms close to your chest, press *hard* several times. Stretch your arms straight in front of you, then over your head, then drop them in front of your abdomen, and repeat the palm pressure. Work up daily to 10 or 20 times in each position.

## VITAMIN E AND SKIN

Q. You have stated that puncturing a vitamin E capsule and rubbing it on the skin had improved the skin of a few who were experimenting with it. Has this continued to be helpful?—P.M., Milltown, New Jersey

A. Yes, it has. But some of the experimenters reported

added improvement by using vitamin A, too. They punctured a 25,000 unit capsule of natural vitamin A and rubbed it on the skin before applying the contents of the 200 I.U. vitamin E capsule. The vitamin A, derived from fish oil, may make you smell a bit fishy, but who cares if it makes you more beautiful?

## DEPILATORIES

Q. What safeguards should one use in regard to depilatories? Are these products dangerous when applied to under-arms?—B.P.J., Seattle, Washington

A. To get help with the question on depilatories, I wrote to Irwin I. Lubowe, M.D., an internationally recognized dermatologist. Here is his response: "Depilatories contain a chemical which may cause irritation when used under the arm, especially after shaving. Occasionally we see an allergic reaction manifested by redness and inflammation. It is advisable to wash away the residual depilatory with a neutral soap. Then cover the area with a thin film of soothing cream. This will reduce the irritation."

## TAPEWORMS

Q. Can you give me any remedy for tapeworms in both animals and people? My veterinarian has given up on my dog, and I have a friend who has had a diagnosis of tapeworm but nothing has helped.—A.J.W., La Mirada, California

A. I found a suggestion from a doctor in an unpublished manuscript. He said that though many doctors have their patients fast for a day or so before giving them a tapeworm medicine, he personally believed that because it is a parasite, a tapeworm cannot be successfully starved. Instead, he had good results by feeding his patients foods for a day or two, which tapeworms do not like: Onions, garlic, pickles and salted fish. He found that these foods tend to weaken the worm, cause it to lose its grip, and thus be expelled more easily when the medicine is finally taken.

A great believer in herbs, the doctor states that taking

a strong tea of walnut leaves (available in the herb tea section in health stores) has removed millions of tapeworms and other parasites. He suggested making a strong infusion of the leaves and refrigerating it. He recommended a wineglass of it several times daily for adults, and an occasional teaspoon or tablespoon for children, according to age. He did not say how to use it for animals.

For the usual parasites, I have witnessed good results from raw garlic, minced, and embedded in a small raw hamburger ball (so the dog will not notice it). People, including children, have also had good results when all other remedies failed by swallowing minced raw garlic followed by fruit juice, or taking garlic perles (from health stores). This, however, is for ordinary worms, not tapeworms.

Remember, after *any* vermifuge is taken, if it is not repeated within two weeks, and several times later, an entire colony of parasites can develop from a few eggs which may be, and usually are, left behind after the worming process.

## NYLON ALLERGY

Q. My sister is allergic to nylon. For about two years I have been trying to find out if there is any place pantyhose of silk or cotton can be purchased. Do you know of any concern which makes such products? I have found none. Also, I have heard that nylon stockings prevent adequate circulation of air to the feet. I would appreciate any help you can give.—A.R.D., Newsome, Virginia

A. Allergy to nylon is not unusual. It is fortunate that your sister has discovered the cause of her allergy. I have a friend who is allergic to wool; she breaks out in a rash whenever she wears it, but it took much trial and error for her to learn the cause.

## BATH PRODUCTS

Q. I am a slightly perplexed man who needs information. First, I understand that there are products available to improve one's bath. What are they? Second, I am supposed to eat a raw egg in milk, also oatmeal. What is so good about raw eggs and oatmeal? If I knew what they contained maybe I could take them in supplement form, and satisfy my needs more easily—H.B., Wautoma, Wisconsin

A. There are many things you can add to bath water. You can buy a mineral product in health stores, or you can add some sea water. (Be sure it comes in filtered form from a health store or from mid-ocean to avoid pollution contamination.) You can add Epsom salts, which are said to help draw out poisons in the body. Or you can add essence of pine (preferably natural, not synthetic) in some form. Epsom salts and natural pine essence are available in drug stores. You can add apple cider vinegar to help your skin maintain its natural acidity. Or you can put some oatmeal in a little bag and swish it in the water, for smoother skin. There is a never-ending list of herbs and other substances to try.

Eggs are considered a nearly perfect food. The biological value is so high (0.94) that egg protein is used as a standard for judging the value of other proteins. Furthermore, except for those few who are allergic to eggs, they are so easily digested that they are completely absorbed by the gastrointestinal tract. (*American Journal of Clinical Nutrition,* May, 1968)

Animal trainers feed raw eggs to priceless pets or show animals to give gloss to their coats. There is objection by some investigators to feeding raw egg whites to human beings, since many people seem to be intolerant of the whites. According to one physician, this is because in *in*fertile egg whites, the important amino acid, cystine, is unavailable to the body. However, in *fertile* eggs, cystine is available and thus the white can be tolerated. Fertile eggs also contain lecithin, an emulsifier for cholesterol.

Fertile eggs are laid by hens raised on the ground where they can peck and eat under natural conditions. A rooster is also present. Thus, fertile eggs hatch.

Infertile eggs, from hens raised in cages without a rooster, do not hatch. Fertile eggs must have the life-giving elements to nourish the baby chicks. Produced according to nature, rather than by mechanized methods, fertile eggs have darker yolks, firmer whites, and contain more vitamins and minerals. They are a food which is hard to beat.

Oatmeal is another valuable food. A study conducted long ago with elderly people proved this. The subjects were fed a breakfast food of nearly raw oatmeal (covered with boiling water in the bowl for a few minutes to soften but not cook it) plus grated apple and chopped nuts, and this brought a health improvement within six weeks. The Scotch and Welsh people have long made oatmeal their staple food. Oatmeal contains protein; B vitamins thiamin, riboflavin, niacin, pantothenic acid and choline; vitamin E; calcium; phosphorous; iron; copper; and silicon.

A silicon deficiency may cause skin and muscle flabbiness, fatigue and dull hair and eyes.

Be sure to purchase steel-cut oats at a health food store. This type of oatmeal has not been robbed of important nutrients by the milling and refining process.

These whole, natural foods are a more complete source of nutrients, and certainly cheaper than many supplements, which may be synthetic and may not contain all of the same nutrients. Whoever recommended these foods to you gave you good advice.


## HEXACHLOROPHENE

Q. Is it true that most deodorants contain hexachlorophene, which Ralph Nader calls dangerous?—E.G., Staten Island, New York


A. Not only have underarm deodorants been found to contain hexachlorophene, but the new, highly advertised vaginal deodorants contain it, too. Furthermore, according to the *New York Times* (Dec. 7, 1971), hexachlorophene is found in some 300 to 400 other products in general use. These include soaps, shampoos, foot powders, baby lotions, shoe liners, household detergents, mouthwash, cosmetics, toothpastes, throat lozenges, sun tan lotion and a burn treatment. It has also been accepted for use on citrus fruits and many vegetables, including cucumbers, peppers, tomatoes and potatoes.

Is hexachlorophene really dangerous? A famed medical center reports six cases of brain seizure in babies (it is used on newborn infants in hospitals), and it has been implicated in the death of adults by a medical society. Adults who use hexachlorophene products in the shower have been found with blood levels of nearly one-third of that which caused brain damage in rats, whereas the highest level of hexachlorophene found in a baby was more than half that in rats.

In adults, this preparation has caused skin darkening as well as dermatitis resulting from skin exposure to sunlight following its use. The American Academy of Pediatrics has warned: "In substantial dosage, hexachlorophene is neurotoxic in rats and has caused the death of a toddler . . . Deaths have also been caused when the chemical was absorbed after application to badly burned skin of children and adults." A reader wrote me that her husband became bald after using a "deodorant soap" on his head whenever he showered.

Dr. Francis N. Marzulli, chief of the FDA Dermal (skin) Toxicity Branch, said: "We know that hexachlorophene can get into the body very easily . . . we also knew previously that it would be toxic if ingested through the mouth or injected into the body. But then we did not suspect it might be hazardous in other ways."

Certainly, applied in underarm and vaginal deodorants, the chemical has easy access to the body through the delicate membranes, despite the claims by manufacturers of such products that "there is no danger." Recent epidemics of skin diseases across the nation followed findings in 2,300 cases by allergy specialists who pinpointed the deodorants which contained hexachlorophene as the culprits. Dr. James F. Molloy, writing in the *Journal of the American Medical Association,* reported dozens of cases of serious skin diseases in a Southern state less than a month after a deodorant soap was introduced in that area. Dr. John L. Morse, a New York dermatologist, cited the reactions of 186 patients: "Some had itching and a burning sensation, others a stinging sensation, and a number developed a redness . . ."

Some deodorants contain a form of aluminum which has also caused toxicity in cases which were confirmed by the user's physicians. Can you tell by the label if these chemicals are included in a deodorant? Not necessarily. Sometimes they appear on a label, but in the case of cosmetics (which may include deodorants), the law does not require the label to state ingredients.

# NUTRITION AND DISEASE

Q. My husband is hypochondriac. He takes a pill for everything. I tell him that his sickness is all in his mind. Don't you think I'm right?—A.D., Chicago, Illinois

A. Yes and no. It depends on what kind of pills he takes. If they are nutritional supplements, that's one thing. But if they are tranquilizers, pep pills and other drugs, which he takes indiscriminately, then that's an entirely different matter.

It is true that the mind can play a lot of tricks on us. A study conducted in the U.S. reported that 85 patients admitted to a hospital for a variety of physical complaints were suffering from depression in disguise. Dr. Hans Selye, revered internationally for his work, discovered that stress can cause physical disease. He proved it with animals, as shown in a movie he made of his findings. The reason stress causes disease is that if you live in constant fear, dread, anxiety, resentment or worry, you constrict, perhaps unconsciously, many of your body functions. Circulation is cut off to various organs—the organ affected differs in different people—and disease can eventually follow in those areas.

If the body is suffering from nutritional deficiencies, pill-popping in the form of natural vitamins—added to a rich nutritional diet—can be condoned. But drugs may be only a crutch and mask a situation, as aspirin relieves a headache but may not cure the underlying cause. Actually, both the mind and nutrition are involved in maintaining good health, so a constructive program in both directions is indicated.

Q. Is it possible to treat a duodenal ulcer by diet?—G.P., Philadelphia, Pennsylvania

A. A duodenal ulcer patient should be under the care

of a doctor, but if your doctor has not already seen it, you might call his attention to a study, "Dietary Treatment in Duodenal Ulcer," conducted at the Iowa Veteran's Administration Hospital by two physicians and a dietitian of the State University of Iowa College of Medicine (reported in *American Journal of Clinical Nutrition,* November, 1969, p. 1536).

Of 103 patients admitted to this study, 50 received bland diets and 53 received regular diets. The age range was from 32 to 79 years. The bland diet was nutritionally high and excluded fried foods, highly seasoned foods, raw fruits (except ripe bananas), food with seeds or tough skin and all raw vegetables. Milk and antacids were added for both bland and regular diets. The regular diet was planned to meet the nutritional requirements of normal, healthy people. There were no restrictions as to type of food or method of preparation.

Although discomfort followed the intake of a few food items on the regular diet (sauerkraut was the main offender) many patients on the regular diet were pleasantly surprised and relieved when they found they could eat the non-bland foods without difficulty.

The authors of this study reported their surprising results: "Clinical response and rate of healing of duodenal ulcer *were the same in both groups.* Our data lead us to believe that duodenal patients do not ordinarily need restricted diets."

Q. How does a calcium deficiency cause constipation and muscle spasms? How can I balance my calcium intake to control this condition?—Mrs. H.E.K., Battle Lake, Minnesota

A. Spastic constipation, which derives its name from spasms in the large intestine, is caused by a deficiency of several nutrients, not just calcium alone. Many people, for example, have become frightened when leaning over to get a sharp spasm or cramp below the chest area. They immediately fear they are having a heart attack, whereas it was merely a muscle cramp or spasm. Sometimes, several fingers of one hand suddenly become cramped or the muscles of the feet or calves or the legs experience an excruciating spasm or cramp, usually at night. This is similar to what happens in the intestinal muscles. The cause *may* be due to a lack of calcium. Calcium acts as a relaxer, thus an antidote for that muscle cramp or spasm wherever it may occur in the body.

The amount of calcium varies from person to person, but that is not the whole story. Many people take calcium and do not digest it or utilize it. Some vitamin D, some vitamin F (as in unsaturated oils) and of greatest importance, hydrochloric acid, are all necessary to break down the calcium so that the body can use and assimilate it. Taking enough calcium plus the utilizers mentioned above should help the problem. Yogurt, which contains calcium and acid for its digestion as well as for improving the intestinal flora, is an excellent help.

John M. Ellis, M.D., has found that vitamin B-6 relieves the excruciating cramps which occur at night in the calves of the legs, so a deficiency of B-6 might also be a factor in spastic constipation. Potassium (from raw green foods, either in salads or juices) may help, and magnesium is also a muscle relaxer. Be SURE, however, that you take magnesium *between* meals, since at least two kinds of magnesium, dolomite and magnesium oxide are *ant*acids, which help to cancel out the stomach acid needed to digest calcium.

Q. I have recently discovered through tests that I have a serious allergy to all grain products, including buckwheat and yeast. I have not been able to take a B complex nor an E supplement since they are usually derived from yeast, rice polishings, and wheat germ. Is there a company which makes natural organic supplements for allergic persons?—M.L.L., Brooklyn, New York

A. You have a real problem and it may help to know that you are not alone. Many, many people are allergic to grain products, although very few to the right type of brewer's yeast grown on molasses and other goodies instead of waste products. This good type of yeast is known as the *Saccharomyces cerevisiae* species and occurs in a few commercial yeasts in health stores. Many people believe they are allergic to yeast because they suffer from gas after taking it, whereas, since it is a protein, they merely need hydrochloric acid in order to digest it. (This has solved the problem for many.) Also, those who are allergic to grains usually have no trouble with rice polishings or brown rice itself.

As for the other grains, particularly wheat, many bread eaters are allergic to such products and do not know what is causing their trouble. I just recently became aware of unsuspected allergy to wheat germ, wheat germ oil and vitamin E derived from it, in several people who did not dream that these foods were the cause of their palpitations. I wrote Dr. Wilfrid E. Shute, the authority of vitamin E, and he said that formerly they used at their clinic synthetic vitamin E only and that it was still available. Synthetic vitamin E has never seen wheat germ and has proved to be satisfactory for those who are allergic to wheat products.

Q. Both my husband and I have a tendency toward kidney stones. Even if they are removed by surgery, more follow. Is there anything we can do to prevent them?—B.H., Chicago, Illinois

A. Magnesium has been found to aid in protection against kidney stones. H. E. Sauberlich, M.D., of the Army's Fitzsimmons General Hospital, Denver, prescribed a 420 mg. tablet of magnesium oxide daily (to provide 250 mg. of magnesium ion) to patients with kidney stones. As long as this therapy was continued (which had extended to two years when the study was reported), the patients remained free of kidney stones. There were no side effects of the magnesium.[1]

Recent information points out that magnesium is an antacid. Ralph Pressman, Ph.D., states that dolomite, a source of both calcium and magnesium, is a type of rock, ground into a powder, and is not readily soluble in the stomach unless there is a normal supply of gastric juice.[2] For this reason, several reputable companies who provide magnesium in supplement form, either label it as an antacid or state on the label that it should be taken *before* or *between* meals so as not to interfere with the body's digestive acid.

Another finding results from a recent study of babies in an area of Thailand, where kidney stones are common. The study suggests that protein malnutrition may contribute to the development of kidney stones.[3]

In connection with the use of magnesium, recent reports reveal that whereas some people do not assimilate magnesium oxide or dolomite properly, they seem to assimilate magnesium alginate, derived from kelp, with no difficulty. Even so, the label suggests taking this form of magnesium before a meal.

Magnesium is a mineral which is growing in importance and apparently has been long overlooked. Many Americans are deficient in magnesium, a lack of which can cause, in addition to kidney stones, heart and prostate disturbance, nervousness and irritability, leg cramps, hand tremor, as well as aching neck and shoulder muscles, restless eyes and fingers and a fast heartbeat.[4]

1. "The Magic Mineral, Magnesium," Chapter 17, from *Get Well Naturally,* by Linda Clark (available at health stores).
2. "Calcium, the Neglected Mineral," by Ralph Pressman, Ph.D., *National Health Federation Bulletin,* May, 1970, p. 20.
3. *The American Journal of Clinical Nutrition,* July, 1970, p. 941.
4. *Natural Health and World and the Naturopath,* August, 1970, p. 1.

## MIGRAINE HEADACHES

Q. Help! Help! I am a victim of migraine headaches. The doctor gives me caffergot to keep them under control but I have been unable to lick them completely, so I am drug-dependent. I would like to know of a better, natural approach.—E.G., San Francisco, California

A. I have covered the subject of migraines at length in my book, *Get Well Naturally.* There is not space to repeat the information here, but there is one new remedy which has come to my attention since the early editions of the book and I have tried it and passed it on to other former migraine sufferers with great success. This remedy is niacin, a B vitamin. Now listen closely, because I don't want you to be surprised—or frightened—if you take niacin. Niacin is another name for nicotinic acid and when one takes it, there is usually an intense flush which gradually spreads over the body. (There is a product called Niacinamide, with the flushing characteristic removed, but it does not seem to do the job for migraines.) This flush lasts about 15 minutes, during which time you turn beet red, but, if the niacin is used according to the proper dosage as recommended by an M.D., there is no danger at all—just temporary discomfort, far less disturbing than the long drawn out migraine itself.

A migraine, as every victim knows, usually starts with peculiar symptoms—a partial, temporary blocking of vision, flashes of light, or spots before the eyes; later followed by excruciating pain and nausea. In the book by Lewis J. Silvers, M.D., *Doctor Silvers' Extraordinary Remedies and Prescriptions for Health and Longevity* (Prentice Hall, Englewood Cliffs, N.J., 1964), the migraine remedy is given. He says, "At the very first symptoms, even if they awaken you out of a deep sleep, immediately take 50 mg. of Niacin (available at drug or health stores). If a flush ensues, the dose is sufficient to quickly dilate the constricted cerebral blood vessels. If you do not flush within ten minutes, take another tablet to produce the salutary flush or dilation of the vessels of the skin. Presto—no migraine."

Q. I have a teen-age child whose face is literally covered with warts. The doctor has tried to burn them off—a painful process—but the warts returned. Is there any other remedy that will do the job?—E.D., Monterey, California

A. This condition is unpleasant for anyone, but for a teen-ager, who is already self-conscious and sensitive, it is practically a disaster. A friend of mine with a teen-age son had the same condition. They, too, tried medical methods with no lasting results. Finally in desperation the father remembered a natural remedy used by his grandmother: castor oil. So the boy's parents asked him to rub castor oil on the warts each night before bedtime and suggested that he try to sleep on his back so as not to rub off the oil on the pillow. Within two weeks the warts had all disappeared and have not returned. There are no scars on his skin, either. He, as well as the parents, are overjoyed.

Q. Japanese doctors treating Parkinson's Disease with the drug L-Dopa found that this product, which I understand is an amino acid, has grown hair. What foods is this substance found in?—C.C.A., Kent, Washington

A. L-Dopa is developed from the horse bean, "viscis fabia." Although it has been reported to bring dramatic relief to sufferers of Parkinson's Disease, high dosages are required and side effects—such as occasional nausea, dizziness, and gastro-intestinal disturbances—have been noted. Parkinson's Disease is a disturbance marked by tremors, muscle rigidity and loss of speech and coordination. Dopamine is naturally found in the body, and of which Parkinsonism apparently indicates a deficiency. L-Dopa is now being synthesized. An amino acid is a protein factor and possibly accompanies the other amino acids in proteins, though I have not seen this explained, nor in what other foods, if any, it is found. I would say that the drug, available by prescription only, is a risky way to grow hair.

Q. I read with concern that, judging by tests on American G.I.'s in Vietnam, most Americans, including young children, are afflicted with varying degrees of hardening of the arteries. Isn't there some simple thing that we can do to prevent heart disease which may be a result of this disturbance?—Mrs. J. deV., Chicago, Illinois

A. Of course there are various types and causes of heart disease. Doctor John Yudkin, of England, has pointed an accusing finger at one culprit in heart disease: sugar. Cutting down on sweets would help to satisfy this requirement. This does *not* mean to substitute artificial sweeteners. It means to really overcome that sweet tooth, which can be done. The more sugar one eats, the more one wants; the less one eats the less one wants. You can gradually cut down sweets in your own and your family's diet. A study conducted at Northwestern University School of Medicine showed that patients with coronary heart disease definitely consumed more sugar, drank more coffee and smoked more cigarettes than controls. (*Lancet,* 1968, ii, 1049-51)

Two brother physicians, the Doctors Shute, of Canada, have returned thousands of cases of heart disease to normal living by the use of sufficiently high doses of d-alpha tocopherol, vitamin E. As a result of world-wide documented studies of the effect of vitamin E on the heart, many persons use this vitamin as a preventive for heart disease.

A third method of self-protection has just been reported from the Netherlands Institute of Nutrition (*American Journal of Clinical Nutrition;* November, 1969, p. 1521). A simple method was tried with human beings, ranging in age from four to 91, for maintaining a normal cholesterol. Cholesterol levels rose when butter, or margarines containing 10%, even 30% of polyunsaturated fat, were eaten. But when margarine containing 50%—or over—of polyunsaturated fatty acids was used, the cholesterol became—and remained—normal without any other dietary changes!

Our labels on margarines in this country do not tell us the percentage of polyunsaturated fat. However, many nutritionists believe that there is a simple formula to keep cholesterol from piling up in the body: a daily intake of 1 to 4 tablespoons of lecithin granules a day, depending on the cholesterol level, or a teaspoonful, night and morning, of liquid lecithin. Lecithin is a food, not a drug, and therefore completely safe.

Q. About a year ago I changed my diet to include a greater amount of protein and to reduce the amount of starches and sweets. I added all the vitamins, too. My problem is embarrassing: I suffer from much gas. Is it possible to take something which will help my system use protein correctly, since I feel sure that is my trouble? I am sixty years old.—E.M.C.

A. I wish all questions were as easy to answer as this one. At your age, and sometimes even earlier, the manufacture of hydrochloric acid begins to slow down. Protein cannot be digested without a sufficient amount of this stomach acid.

Q. My feet are killing me! I have to stand on them all day long
and when I get home at night, I actually cry because my feet
hurt and my whole body aches. Please help!—M.S., Croton-on-
Hudson, New York

A. I know what you mean. When your feet hurt, you
hurt all over. Furthermore, pinched, hurting feet can
make lines in your face from the strain they inflict.
Watch any woman who has been shopping for several
hours in high heels hunting for a place to sit down so
that she can kick off her shoes. And look at her face.
You will see all the discomfort registered there.

Fortunately, we are beginning to live in a period of
emancipation and shoes are now available which pamper
your feet even though they don't look like the conven-
tional shoes men and women have worn for centuries.
There are several choices: The custom-made shoe to
fit your own foot. It takes many weeks of waiting until
they are ready and they are expensive. Still, many people
believe they are worth it since they undoubtedly bring
blessed relief. You can usually find a source in the yellow
pages of your phone book.

There is a new Scandinavian shoe, selling for less than
$10, which is now appearing in shoe shops in nearly
every American town and city. The soles are made of
wood and the flexible top is perforated with small holes.
These have also brought relief to men and women who
say they can stand in them for hours without discomfort.

But my favorite is a sandal which is heavenly to wear.
It is more expensive than the Scandinavian "clogs," but
still very inexpensive in comparison to the space shoe.
These sandals are made in Germany, and are the next
best thing to walking barefoot. The inside sole is built
to support and cuddle your feet, your arches, and give
freedom to your toes, exactly as your foot makes a
footprint on wet sand. All of us who wear them, women
and men, swear by them and can walk or stand in them
for hours without foot fatigue or nervous exhaustion.
If your arch is too flat, it helps correct it. One woman
found she could later wear a half-size shorter in a dress
shoe after wearing these sandals. If your arch is too

high, they help this problem, too. You must, however, allow about two weeks to become accustomed to wearing the sandals. One man reported that after wearing them, his backache vanished. A woman said her headaches ceased. Both cases may have been due to corrected posture, which the sandals promote, or to relief from pinched, squeezed and distorted nerves of the feet which can radiate pain all over the body. Still another woman lost a growth on the bottom of her foot which had defied all other treatment.

At first, any of these unconventional shoes may look strange to you. But when you trade them for comfort, you learn to love them. At the moment, they come in only one color, but they can be dyed.

Such shoes which allow the feet to be comfortable are now "in." So you need suffer no longer.

Q. My husband, who is over sixty, had a heart attack over a year ago. Because he will not, or cannot stop smoking, I am afraid he is going to have another. We have been married only a short time and I do not want to lose him! His doctor has told him to quit and I have done everything I know. He takes all supplements, eats an excellent diet and gets good outdoor exercise. He is doing wonderfully well, but I am afraid it can't last as long as he continues smoking. Can you help me?—N.S. (No Address).

A. I will give you the steps in a new method which claims one can stop smoking and lose all desire to smoke. William P. Knowles, an English expert on breathing, says that of students from 100 countries, eight out of 10 have stopped smoking entirely or greatly reduced their intake. A secretary who smoked 25 cigarettes daily, suffered from bronchitis and a cough, stopped smoking in two months, after taking the course two years ago. Recently she tried a cigarette to test herself; the taste, she said, was awful. "My desire to smoke is gone, along with the bronchitis and the cough."

Before I go on, let me make a suggestion. It is important to discover why a person is a compulsive smoker. It might be due to hypoglycemia (low blood sugar). It may be habit or insecurity. It may be an attempt to relieve stress. If you are making him uncomfortable about his smoking, you may be doing him more harm than the smoking. Relax. Take an "I don't care" attitude. Tell him about the new method which follows, but don't push or nag. There is more than one way of losing a husband, even though from the best intentions. Here are the steps of the Knowles system. It is done three time daily, for three minutes each.

1. Sit upright in a chair. Don't touch the back of the chair with your spine.

2. Stretch your arms forward, then draw them back slowly; let your elbows rest against the sides of your body; put hands—palms down—on your thighs.

3. Breathe in and out quickly through your nose about a dozen times. A smoker may cough and sputter, but this is good for expelling phlegm and stale air.

4. Once the lungs are cleansed, exhale slowly and completely until there is no air left in your lungs. Then inhale to the count of seven. Pause for one second, exhale. Do this breathing 14 times, seven in and seven out. Keep your chest out and shoulders back to allow freedom for breathing. That's it!

## Six New Books To Make You
## FEEL BETTER . . . LOOK BETTER . . .
## NATURALLY!

☐ **FOOD ADDITIVES AND YOUR HEALTH** by Beatrice Trum Hunter. An original book by the author of **The Natural Foods Cookbook.** The dangers of commercial additives—how to avoid them and choose your food wisely. (95¢)

☐ **BETTER FOOD FOR BETTER BABIES** by Gena Larson. An original book with many recipes—an inspiring guidebook by one of the most respected names in the nutrition field. (95¢)

☐ **FACT/BOOK ON VITAMINS & OTHER FOOD SUPPLE-MENTS** by Carlson Wade. Factual, practical, the answers to the questions most people have about this vital health area. (95¢)

☐ **YOUR BODY IS YOUR BEST DOCTOR** by Melvin E. Page, D.D.S. and H. Leon Abrams, Jr. Startling information on health, body chemistry and nutrition and a revolutionary program for natural health. ($1.25)

☐ **LIGHT ON YOUR HEALTH PROBLEMS** by Linda Clark. Answers to the most frequently asked questions about health, vitamins and natural beauty care—from her famous column in **Let's LIVE** magazine. ($1.25)

☐ **NATURAL FOODS BLENDER COOKBOOK** by Frieda Nusz. A unique two-in-one cookbook—a healthful collection of more than 200 blender-made dishes and drinks you can whip up in minutes. ($1.25)

**Buy them at your local bookstore or use this handy coupon**

---

**Keats Publishing Inc. Dept. 2**　　　　　　　　　　　　H-100
**212 Elm St., New Canaan, Conn. 06840**

Please send me the books checked above. I am enclosing

$_________________. (Check or money order—no currency, no C.O.D.'s please. If less than 4 books, add 25¢ per book for postage and handling. We pay postage on 5 books or more). Please allow up to three weeks for delivery.

Name_______________________________________________

Address____________________________________________

City________________________State__________Zip________

(2)